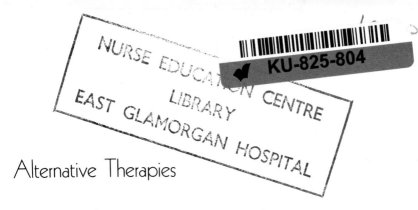
Alternative Therapies

Alternative Therapies

A Guide to Complementary Medicine for the Health Professional

Edited by

G. T. Lewith, MA, MRCP, MRCGP

Co-Director, The Centre for the Study of Alternative Therapies, Southampton

William Heinemann Medical Books
London

First published 1985
by William Heinemann Medical Books Ltd,
23 Bedford Square,
London WC1B 3HH

© G. T. Lewith, 1985

ISBN 0–433–19270–4

Photoset and printed in Great Britain by
Redwood Burn Limited, Trowbridge, Wiltshire and
bound by Pegasus Bookbinding, Melksham, Wiltshire

Contents

Contributors

H. Boyd MB, CHB, FRCP, DCH, FFHOM.
Consultant Physician, Glasgow Homoeopathic Hospital,
Glasgow

J. Kenyon MD, MB, CHB
Co-Director, The Centre for the Study of Alternative Therapies,
Southampton

G. T. Lewith MA, MRCP, MRCGP
Co-Director, The Centre for the Study of Alternative Therapies,
Southampton

D. Marcer BSC, PHD
Senior Lecturer, Department of Psychology,
University of Southampton, Southampton

P. Wells BA, MCSP, DIPTP
Superintendent Physiotherapist, St Stephen's Hospital, London

Preface

Over the last two or three years many articles and papers have been published in both the lay and medical press about various alternative therapies. Some authors have suggested that 'belief' in a therapy is adequate proof of its efficacy. Others have adopted an equally irrational stance of 'non-belief', whatever the evidence provided. In spite of our current academic inquisitive and apparently open-minded attitudes to health, the bulk of medical opinion staggers on regardless of the issues and opinions it chooses not to consider and the evidence it chooses not to accept. The exception being information that substantiates the currently held 'acceptable' opinions. It appears to me that this situation has remained unchanged for centuries as it has always been difficult to introduce new ideas into essentially conservative and protectionist professional organisations.

I have strived to achieve some balance within this book and have attempted to provide a forum in which some of the more important areas of the medical alternatives can be considered rationally. The aim of this text is to inform those within the medical and paramedical professions about these therapies, how they might work, and whom they might benefit. Information about reputable bodies concerned with practice and teaching within these areas is appended to the end of each chapter.

Western medicine has devoted an enormous amount of time, energy and money investigating body structure. We now have at our disposal excellent scanning techniques, which provide us with an enormous amount of information. Even some of the methods available that attempt to measure body function, such as liver function tests, do little more then tell us about the death of liver tissue. We have no real method for assessing whether the liver is stressed and about to undergo structural change. Furthermore, many of our methods of assessing therapies are based on looking at large populations in order to evaluate the effect of a particular treatment.

Western medicine does not really allow the enquiring doctor to ask specific questions about the origin of a particular disease in an individual. It is possible that common diseases, such as rheumatoid arthritis, can be caused by any one of perhaps 40 or 50 stimuli, and the disease complex of rheumatoid arthritis represents the body's reaction, in susceptible individuals, to any one of these triggers.

The conceptual and philosophical models used in alternative medicine attempt to arrive at a causal diagnosis for a patient's complaint, offering treatment at a causal level. For instance, the treatment of rheumatoid arthritis with homoeopathy may in some instances be directed at the treatment of chronic streptococcal infections, while in other instances the apparent trigger may be insecticide poisoning.

All the alternative medicines have as their basis some concept which involves biological energy or vital force. The homoeopath or acupuncturist considers that disturbances in the body's energetic balance represent the first stage of a disease process and that structural change is a secondary phenomenon. Many of the alternative therapies are therefore directed at normalising the body's own energy, rather than simply dealing with organic changes. At the present time we are unsure about the validity of many of these conceptual models and far more research will be required before we can make any real effort to evaluate them objectively.

I helped to establish the Centre for the Study of Alternative Therapies in Southampton, in the profound belief that treatments such as acupuncture and homoeopathy have much to offer mankind and that research and education within these areas were both essential and long overdue. At the centre we practise a range of therapies and attempt to provide a very broad-base (conventional and alternative) approach to health care and disease prevention. I hope this eclecticism is reflected in the critical but open-minded attitudes to the various therapies discussed in this text. It seems to me that some of the more exciting and potentially useful concepts within medicine exist in the philosophies of the various alternative therapies. Many of these ideas will prove to be false, but if some could be verified and formulated in a more specific and practical manner, then we might reap untold rewards which at present elude our current approaches to health and disease.

G. T. Lewith   Southampton, 1985

Chapter 1

Acupuncture and transcutaneous nerve stimulation (TENS)

G. T. Lewith

Introduction

This chapter is designed to provide the reader with an overall view of acupuncture and transcutaneous electrical nerve stimulation (TENS). The majority of the information is devoted to acupuncture, and covers both the historical and philosophical aspects of this treatment as well as the more scientific evidence available from neurophysiological studies and controlled clinical trials. My aim is not to provide instruction about the practice of acupuncture, but rather to inform the reader about how this therapy may be effective and in what conditions, and under what situations, it would be best for patients to seek acupuncture treatment. The short section on TENS is more practical, and is designed to inform those in the medical and paramedical fields about the use of this treatment in the context of day-to-day clinical practice. A list of further reading is appended to this chapter for those interested as well as information about how to obtain and study acupuncture therapy.

The development of Chinese medicine

Acupuncture (or needle puncture) is a European term invented by Willem Ten Rhyne, a Dutch physician who visited Nagasaki in Japan in the early part of the seventeenth century. The Chinese describe acupuncture by the character 'Chen', which literally means 'to prick with a needle'.

Acupuncture has a recorded history of about 2000 years, but some authorities claim that it has been practised in China for much longer. The Chinese believe that stone knives or sharp-edged tools were used some 4000 years ago to puncture and drain abscesses; these instruments were called 'Bian' stones. The character 'Bian' means the use of a sharp-edged stone to treat disease. The modern Chinese character 'Bi' describes a disease of pain and is almost certainly derived from the use of 'Bian' stones for the treatment of painful complaints.

The origin of Chinese medicine is a complex story, and acupuncture represents only one facet of the development of the Chinese medical system. The first recorded attempt at conceptualising and treating disease dates back to about 1500 BC; tortoise shells with inscriptions dating from that time were thought to have been used for divination and also in the art of healing. The philosophical basis for much of very early Chinese medicine seems to have been to seek harmony between the living and their dead ancestors, and the good and evil spirits that inhabited the earth.

The first known acupuncture text is the *Nei Ching Su Wen*. This book is also known by a variety of alternative titles such as the *Yellow Emperor's Classic of Internal Medicine*, or the *Canon of Medicine*. The initial section of the *Nei Ching Su Wen* involves a discussion between the Yellow Emperor, Huang Ti, and his Minister, Ch'i Pai, which lays down the philosophical framework of traditional Chinese medical thought. The authorship of the *Nei Ching Su Wen* is attributed to Huang Ti, but there is some doubt as to whether he actually existed and a great deal more uncertainty as to who wrote the book. It was probably written by a variety of people and seems to date from the Warring States period (475–221 BC).

The Western doctor observes the facts before him and uses the current physiological theories to explain them. Chinese medicine is based on a much wider world view, but one that is more difficult to justify and almost impossible to test within the context of an empirical experiment. These ideas are woven into a complete system based on a philosophy different from that of Western medicine; for instance, the concept of Yin and Yang and the number 5 are two of the more important factors permeating much of traditional Chinese scientific thought.

The Warring States period is a particularly interesting time in Chinese history and has exerted a great deal of influence on Chinese thought. Two main philosophical ideologies emerged during this time, Taoism and Confucianism. Confucianism defined the social status of prince and pauper within Chinese society and elected the Emperor a god. It resulted in a basically feudal and totalitarian system of government that exists today in an adapted form. Taoism represented quite a different approach; the Tao literally means the 'way' and the philosophy of Taoism is a method of maintaining harmony between man and his world, and between this world and beyond. The Taoist concept of health is to attempt to attain perfect harmony between the opposing forces of the natural world—between Yin and Yang—the belief being that the only way to be healthy is to adjust to these natural forces and become part of their rhythm. Furthermore, such forces are completely dependent on each other: earth is dependent on rain and rain is dependent on heaven, which in turn cannot exist without earth. The concept of a unified, but at the same time polar, force governing natural events is central to much of Chinese scientific thought.

At first glance these concepts seem to be an irrelevant sideline to the development of a system of medicine, but acupuncture as practised by the ancient Chinese can only really be understood if the reader grasps the traditional Chinese approach to health and disease. In essence the ideal of health is perfect harmony between the forces of Yin and Yang. However, this state is rarely attained and most of us exist in a state of fluctuating health: one day we feel well and the next day less well. The Western doctors' concept of a healthy patient (which is usually primarily based on normal examination and investigation) is an anathema to traditional Chinese thought. All of us are in a state of change, but it is only when this change causes persistent and irreversible disharmony that it results in established disease.

Acupuncture needles and moxibustion

As acupuncture developed, the Bian stones were discarded and needles of stone and pottery were developed. Eventually metal needles appeared, and these took the form of the classical 'nine needles', each with a different function—a sort of Chinese physician's surgical kit. The main needle now used for acupuncture is the filliform (Fig. 1.1), as most of the others have been replaced by more sophisticated surgical instruments such as scalpels or forceps.

A discussion of the development of acupuncture is incomplete without mentioning moxibustion. This is the burning on or near the skin of the herb moxa. The Chinese character 'Chiu' is used

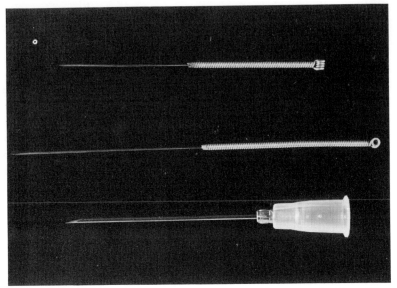

Fig. 1.1 *A 1 inch and a 1½ inch acupuncture needle compared with an 18 gauge injection needle.*

to describe the art of moxibustion, and literally means 'to scar with a burning object'. Moxibustion does not now involve scarring, but moxa is still used to provide local heat over acupuncture points. It is made from the dried leaves of *Artemisia vulgaris* and the Chinese believe that the older the moxa the better its therapeutic properties.

The evolution of acupuncture points and channels

Acupuncture points are undoubtedly the end-product of millions of detailed observations and, as they were developed, so each of them was given a Chinese name which implied its functional and clinical importance. There is an instinctive urge to cause more pain over a painful area; the image of a person with toothache pressing on the painful tooth is a frequent cartoonist's joke. As Melzack has demonstrated, common painful diseases consistently cause painful points to emerge in well-defined anatomical locations. When such a point is stimulated, the pain can be alleviated, hence the idea of a point for treating pain. From this simple beginning it is easy to see how a system of acupuncture points evolved for the management of painful conditions.

Acupuncture points were subsequently grouped into a system of channels which run over the body (Fig. 1.2); the channels are said to conduct the flow of vital energy through the body. Furthermore, each channel, or group of acupuncture points, was designated with the name of an organ and said to represent the functional integrity of that organ. The Chinese believed that if an organ was malfunctioning, then this would lead to an abnormal flow of vital energy in the channel representing that organ. The therapeutic implication of these assumptions is that the judicious selection of acupuncture points on the appropriate channels could then be used to normalise the flow of vital energy within them and subsequently return the organ to normal function.

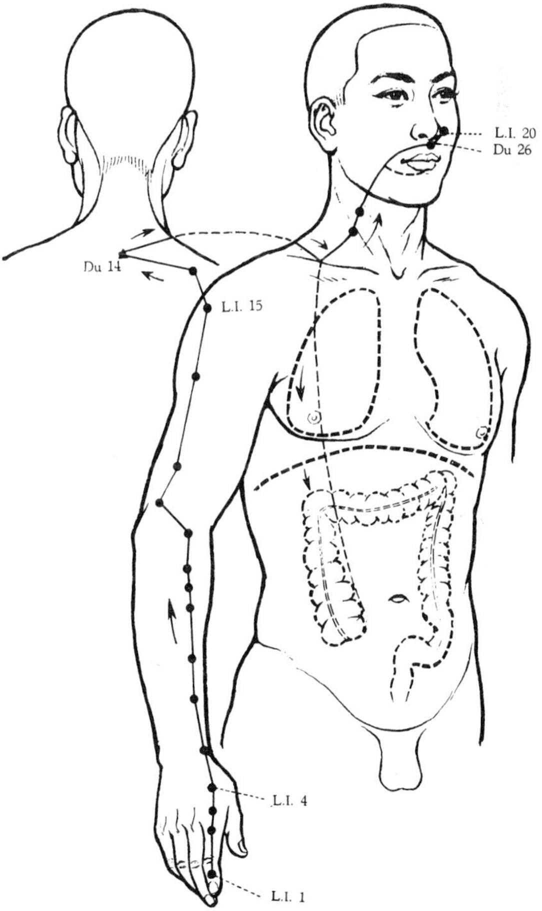

Fig. 1.2 The large intestine channel.

It is almost impossible to understand how this very complex and tautological series of assumptions evolved. However, it does provide a framework which allows the acupuncturist to understand and select points for the treatment of a variety of internal diseases such as asthma and irritable bowel syndrome.

Subsequent development

Over the ensuing centuries, acupuncture and moxibustion became part of a sophisticated medical system. Medical colleges were established in China during the sixth century AD and many well-illustrated and refined texts were published about these therapeutic techniques. During the Ming Dynasty (AD 1368–1644) the first consistent contacts were established with Europe, one of the earliest being in 1504 when the Portuguese landed at Macao. At about the same time, China's fleets began to visit India, Persia and some of the Arab states. With the advent of renewed interest in China, and also the wish of various European nations to 'discover and colonise' the non-European world, the Portuguese began to establish trading settlements in mainland China. With the traders went priests to convert the 'heathen', and it was through these priests, and the various physicians who visited China, that the idea of acupuncture began to filter through to the West. The Jesuits were particularly active in collating and disseminating information, but the process was far from one sided as the Jesuits also introduced Western science to China. Dominique Parrenin, a missionary, translated a textbook of anatomy into Mandarin but this was banned from general circulation by the Emperor as he recognised that many of the Western concepts contradicted those of traditional Chinese medicine.

The Ching Dynasty (AD 1644–1911) was a time of chaos for the Chinese Empire. Western influences pervaded a war-torn China, especially during the nineteenth century when various nations were given spheres of influence on the Chinese mainland. The Ching Emperors regarded acupuncture as a bar to progress, and in 1822 a government decree eliminated acupuncture from the curriculum of the Imperial Medical College.

The art of acupuncture was now in decline. Many acupuncturists seemed to be no more than 'pavement physicians' with poor training. Their surgery was often the market place, their knowledge of traditional Chinese medicine was very limited and their equipment was filthy and of poor quality. The majority of respectable Chinese doctors were practising herbal medicine and massage rather than acupuncture and moxibustion. In spite of its decline, acupuncture remained the medicine of the masses. The Imperial denigration of acupuncture reflected not only the poor standard of practice, but also the fact that some of the educated Chinese were looking to the West for progress.

Western medical colleges were set up by the missionaries, the first being in Canton. The missionaries translated Western medical books into Chinese and in 1886 began to print the *China Medical Missionary Journal* which was the first scientific journal in China. Another medical college was established shortly afterwards in Tientsin and there was a gradual increase in the number of Western-trained Chinese doctors. Finally, in 1929, the practice of acupuncture was outlawed in China; the passage of acupuncture has not always been smooth, even in its homeland!

The recent Chinese enthusiasm for various forms of traditional medicine such as acupuncture was actively cultivated by the Communists. They realised that there were few or no medical services in the 'liberated areas' during the Revolution, and that the traditional methods were cheap and acceptable to the Chinese peasants. Consequently, acupuncture gained new momentum and during the early 1950s many hospitals opened up clinics to provide, teach and investigate the traditional methods of medicine, the main research institutes being in Peking, Shanghai and Nanking. This renaissance of acupuncture combined with a sophisticated scientific approach has allowed the development of many new methods in this therapy and has undoubtedly provided one of the many stimuli for the current Western enthusiasm for the alternative therapies.

Acupuncture in the West

It is probable that acupuncture has been known and used in the West since the seventeenth century, but its first recorded use was by Dr Berlioz at the Paris Medical School in 1810. He treated a young woman suffering from abdominal pain, and although the Paris Medical Society described this as a reckless form of treatment, Dr Berlioz continued to use acupuncture and claimed great success with it.

Acupuncture is not new to England, the first known British acupuncturist being John Churchill who, in 1821, published a series of results on the treatment of tympany and rheumatism with acupuncture. In 1823 acupuncture was mentioned in the first issue of the *Lancet* and in 1824 Dr Elliotson, a physician at St Thomas' Hospital, London, began to use this method of treatment. In 1827 he published a paper describing the treatment of 42 cases of rheumatism by acupuncture, and concluded that this was an effective therapeutic method for such problems.

Ear acupuncture

There are some ancient Chinese manuscripts that mention the use of the external ear for acupuncture, but classical Chinese acupuncture applies to the body rather than the ear. Ear acupuncture has been developed largely outside China and the detailed ear map that is now used by most acupuncturists was developed by Dr Paul Nogier, in France, in the early 1950s.

Ear acupuncture was known to the ancient Egyptians. Ear cauteries have been found in the Pyramids, and these were used for burning or scarring specific ear points for conditions such as sciatica. In 1637 a Portuguese doctor, Zactus Lusitanus, described the use of ear cauteries for sciatica, and in 1717 Valsalva demonstrated the use of ear acupuncture for toothache. These early experiments with ear acupuncture appear to be a separate discovery and to have nothing to do with the growth and development of acupuncture in China. Sciatica seems to have been a problem that was particularly amenable to this form of treatment and studies in the mid-nineteenth century indicate that approximately 60% of people who were treated with ear cautery, for sciatica, obtained relief from their symptoms.

It was this crude form of acupuncture that interested Dr Nogier in the early 1950s. Some of his patients had received ear cautery and obtained relief from pain, and therefore he began to develop and investigate this form of therapy. He produced an ear map (Fig. 1.3), and since the early 1950s he has refined and developed this technique. One of his earliest findings was that if there was pain in the body, then the equivalent part of the ear also became painful. For instance, if the hand is painful then the part of the ear representing the hand also becomes painful when minimal but consistent pressure is applied to the relevant part of

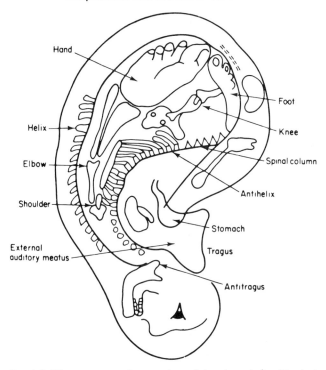

Fig. 1.3 The somatotopic mapping of the pinna (after Nogier).

the pinna. This pain will not be elicited if areas are palpated that represent painless regions of the body. Both the ear map and the assumptions made by Nogier about pain and its treatment have been tested by Oleson *et al.* (1980) in a double-blind manner. A number of patients on an orthopaedic ward were used as subjects and the subsequent results demonstrated that by utilising the ear map, the site of pain could be located in a completely blind manner in over 70% of cases. In view of the technical difficulties involved in such studies, these results are highly significant and imply that Nogier's assumptions are correct.

Painful points

Within the context of Western medicine, the development of acupuncture points on the body demonstrates an interesting story of rediscovery. Over the last 50 years many Western physicians have discovered independently that pressing, stimulating or injecting various superficial body points can help to relieve pain, particularly musculoskeletal pain. These points are not necessarily at the site of pain, but are often at distant areas. For instance, cervical spondylosis frequently presents with pain over the shoulder or scapular region. On close examination, it is frequently possible to define the origin of the pain and demonstrate that the neck is the cause of the problem. However, injection or stimulation of the painful points around the scapula will often relieve the pain and free neck movement. Melzack *et al.* (1977) correlated these trigger points with acupuncture points, and found that most trigger points were already well known and described as acupuncture points. There have been a number of attempts to understand the existence of trigger points, but as yet there is no clear explanation of this phenomenon. It is interesting to note that the Chinese realised this fact some 3000 years ago, and the Ling Shu summarises this approach when it says: 'In pain puncture the tender point'.

Electro-acupuncture

During the 1950s the Chinese began to produce electrical stimulators that allowed a small-amplitude pulsed electrical squarewave to pass between sets of paired acupuncture needles. These were initially used to replace prolonged manual stimulation of acupuncture needles during acupuncture anaesthesia. In the West, such electrical stimulation has frequently been used as part of standard acupuncture therapy, and many of the studies investigating the mechanism of acupuncture and evaluating its clinical effects as an analgesic have used electro-stimulation techniques. Transcutaneous electrical nerve stimulation (TENS) is an adaptation of electro-acupuncture, in that the electrical stimulation is applied through surface electrodes rather than through acupuncture needles.

Most electro-acupuncture stimulators have two main adjustments, frequency and amplitude. The amplitude achieved by these machines is usually fairly small (50 mA into a 1-kΩ load) and the frequency usually varies from 0 to about 2000 Hz. To date, it has been impossible to define the ideal frequencies for individual patients or problems, either for electro-acupuncture or for TENS. However, there has been some suggestion from the studies available that low-frequency stimuli (2–10 Hz) promote the release of the endogenous opiates, and high-frequency stimuli (500–1000 Hz) activate the gating mechanisms and block the onward transmission of pain. But overall not enough is understood about electrical stimulation to give a clear answer as to how it should be best used.

A variety of electrical appliances have been used by acupuncturists to measure and quantify the skin's electrical resistance and conductance over acupuncture points. Becker *et al.* (1976) have demonstrated, within the context of very carefully controlled animal experiments, that acupuncture points have decreased skin resistance as compared with surrounding normal tissue (i.e. they pass electrical current more easily). A number of machines are available which allow the acupuncturist to search the skin for points of increased conductance, the conductance being measured either on a simple resistance meter or by being translated into speaker noise. Within the context of a busy clinical practice, such equipment is particularly prone to artefact as slight alterations in humidity and/or pressure of the probe searching the skin lead to the location of 'false' points. There are over 350 acupuncture points on the body and simply locating them does not really tell the practitioner whether the point requires treatment for a particular patient. Therefore, simple point locators are of limited value, in that they are inaccurate and also fail to provide therapeutically relevant information. Some of the more sophisticated impedence meters available involve far better artefact control. Some of these machines, such as those developed by Dr Voll in West Germany, can be used to measure the charge on acupuncture points very accurately. Voll has suggested that acupuncture points are rather like batteries, and that the charge on a specific point represents the state of health or disease of the point, and the organ or tissue deep in the body which it represents. The Chinese look upon acupuncture points (and channels) as functional representations of the internal organs. Voll has accepted this assumption literally and suggests that if the stomach is diseased, the points on the stomach channel will have altered charge or, more exactly, an altered electromotive force.

By using this more accurate equipment, the acupuncturist can define which points have abnormal electrical readings and can therefore deduce which organs are diseased. Returning the point to a state of normal charge is often enough to control and occasionally cure the internal disease process. There are other systems of acupuncture based on similar principles; Ryodovaku, a Japanese system of acupuncture, is similar to that developed by Voll.

Biologically safe laser beams have also been used to stimulate acupuncture points and therefore to replace acupuncture needles. Some researchers are also interested in the use of magnets and magnetic fields over acupuncture points, but the evaluation of these methods as a form of therapy is fraught with difficulty and very much in its early stages.

Some of the techniques mentioned appear to be both exciting and innovative, and more interestingly because they involve measurement, are open to the type of rigorous scientific experiment which should be able to provide evidence as to their validity. If the assumptions made by Voll and others prove to be correct, particularly with respect to the diagnostic information they provide, then these electro-acupuncture techniques, which are currently in their infancy, will eventually become investigations of enormous value and importance within the context of day-to-day medicine.

Traditional Chinese medicine

While accepting that many doctors practise needle puncture simply by selecting and needling the local tender points which relate to painful areas, it would be inappropriate and historically incorrect to ignore the origins of this system of medicine. Therefore it is important to examine the conceptual and diagnostic systems used within traditional Chinese medicine in order to provide the basis for a more complete understanding of this therapy.

Western medicine presupposes that a human being is Cartesian: the body represents one functioning system and the mind another. It accepts that each system may affect the other, but essentially it sees disease as either physical or mental. The Chinese assume that the body is whole and each part of it is intimately connected, with each organ having a mental as well as a physical function. This perhaps explains why some people see acupuncture as a 'holistic therapy'.

In spite of the current fashionable interest in holism, it is a concept that is almost impossible to define with accuracy. Holism seems to imply a therapy that both treats the patient as a complete functional unit, and can be used to treat almost all conditions from which that patient might suffer. In a diagnostic and conceptual sense, traditional Chinese medicine is holistic as it does assess the patient as a complete functional unit. However, in the therapeutic sense, acupuncture is not holistic; it is one system of treatment and cannot conceivably provide the necessary breadth of therapeutic flexibility required to cure man's ills. Many authors, such as Ivan Illich, have been hypercritical of Western medicine and thus some people have looked upon acupuncture as both an alternative and a superior system of medicine. The major disadvantage of Western medicine is that it has the potential to cause a great deal of harm. Acupuncture, on the other hand, is most unlikely to cause any serious damage as it is a particularly safe form of therapy. This undoubtedly represents a very useful advantage.

Even though the traditional Chinese explanations for acupuncture are somewhat enigmatic to the average Western scientist, acupuncture does seem to have a clearly validated scientific basis with respect to its mechanism of action in painful conditions, as will be discussed in the section on neurophysiology (see page 22. In spite of their radically different philosophical assumptions, it is wiser to look upon Eastern and Western medical systems as mutually beneficial rather than exclusive. Each approach has ideas and therapeutic methods that can be explained both scientifically and philosophically, each can benefit the individual and together they can broaden the philosophical and ideological bases of medicine.

Preventative medicine

The Chinese system of medicine suggests that health is achieved and disease prevented by maintaining the body in a balanced state; this concept could be applied both to individuals and to society as a whole. In individual terms, ancient Chinese physicians preached moderation in all things, such as food and alcohol, and also suggested that normal activities should include mental as well as physical tasks. The wealthier Chinese visited their doctors when they were well, paying a retainer to the doctor as long as they remained healthy; if they became ill, the doctor lost his fee. Such a highly sophisticated and personal system of health care is impractical within our current social and economic environment, but the concept behind these ideas represents the first coherent disease prevention system, designed for the individual.

The cornerstone of health, within the context of traditional Chinese medicine, is a normal fluctuating balance of Yin and Yang. If such balance ceases to exist, then the Chinese believe that external agents (or pathogens) could invade the body and cause disease. The essential principle of traditional Chinese medicine is to specify the exact nature of the imbalance between Yin and Yang, and the pathogen causing the trouble. Acupuncture points can then be selected to correct these pathological processes and, as the natural forces of the body become balanced, the disease will be eliminated. The art of traditional Chinese medicine is to particularise this imbalance accurately so that it can be corrected. The patient is then treated by using specific acupuncture points on the body or ear in order to re-balance the body. In general terms, the patient will give a better response if very few acupuncture points are used, therefore if the acupuncturist can select the appropriate points with accuracy, the patient is likely to show a swift and effective response to treatment.

In allopathic medicine, if a drug is proving ineffective or only partially effective, then, providing no obvious adverse reactions are occurring, it is often legitimate to increase the dose. The treatment of hypertension with gradually increasing doses of a beta-blocker is one example of this general principle. In acupuncture, and indeed within all the alternative therapies, the opposite principle applies. The patient's failure to respond or improve may well suggest that too much therapy has been given. Personal experience also plays an important part in the choice of any particular therapy; most general practitioners know by experience, and from repeated culture and sensitivity results on midstream urine specimens, that ampicillin is a good antibiotic for urinary tract infections. In this instance 'good' means that the urinary tract infection is very likely to resolve within 48 hours and not require any further action. If it fails to resolve within this period of time, the doctor will need to apply his medical training and skill in order to question the diagnosis and, if necessary, work out a more appropriate therapy.

This simple model illustrates many important ideas about point selection in the use of traditional Chinese medicine. Certain acupuncture points seem to be particularly useful for specific conditions; this mirrors very closely the selection of specific antibiotics for common infections. However, if the treatment of choice does not produce an effect, then the therapist must think about the diagnosis with some care and re-evaluate his therapy. Therefore the more the acupuncturist knows about acupuncture, the more likely he is to have therapeutic adaptability within the empirical models of traditional Chinese medicine.

Because these ideas represent general principles they cannot possibly be true in all instances—for example, in many situations the allopathic practitioner will attempt to provide a very accurate and specific therapy—but in general they provide a philosophical basis for contrasting and comparing allopathic medicine with a traditional Chinese approach to health and disease.

The anatomy and physiology of traditional Chinese medicine

The diagnostic and therapeutic principles of Yin and Yang and the pathogens are based on a system of anatomy and physiology peculiar to traditional Chinese medicine. The anatomy of traditional Chinese medicine is represented by the acupuncture points and the channels that connect them. Its physiology has many similarities to that of Western medicine; most of the organ functions defined in the *Nei Ching Su Wen* are accurate in the light of modern scientific discovery.

The heart is said to dominate the circulation of blood. The *Nei Ching* says: 'The heart fills the pulse with blood ... and the force of the pulse flows into the arteries and the force of the arteries ascends into the lungs'. This seems to be a clear description of the double circulation of blood; the idea of blood circulated in this way was peculiar to Chinese medicine until it was 'rediscovered' by William Harvey in the early seventeenth century. The *Nei Ching* also states that the kidneys dominate bone, that they play an integral part in the process of growth and reproduction, and that they control body fluid in concert with the lungs. This represents a series of surprisingly accurate observations in the light of our current thoughts on vitamin D metabolism, the embryological origin of the kidney and gonads, and the detailed and complex systems involved in acid–base balance.

In traditional Chinese medicine the major bodily functions are built around the five main organs—the heart, the lungs, the kidneys, the liver and the spleen. In Western medicine these organs are of vital importance, but not to the same extent as in traditional Chinese medicine. The Chinese call them the five

'Zang' (or solid) organs and it is the system of the five 'Zang' organs that controls the body's health. Each of the 'Zang' (solid) organs is linked to a 'Fu' (hollow) organ. For instance, the kidney is linked both structurally and functionally to the urinary bladder. In Eastern and Western medicine both organs are accepted as controlling the production and passage of urine; the channels representing the kidney and urinary bladder are also paired as vital energy is said to flow from one channel to the other. The liver and gall bladder are linked in a similar manner and it must be apparent that equivalent structural and functional interrelationships for these organs exist within conventional medicine.

The pairing of channels is important when deciding on which acupuncture points should be used; diseases of any organ can be treated by using the paired channel. For example, a liver problem can be treated by using acupuncture points on the gall bladder channel. Traditional Chinese medicine considers migraine to be a disease of the liver and these headaches can therefore be effectively treated by using points on the gall bladder channel.

Traditional Chinese medicine assumes that the emotions are governed by individual organs; it does not consider the brain and subconscious as discrete entities. Therefore the body and mind are a real part of the same functional system. Each organ is given a particular emotion, for instance the liver is said to be the organ affected by anger or irritability. The concept that emotional functions are completely tied in with physical ones is deeply rooted in Chinese culture; there is less stigma attached to the neurotic as they are considered to have a disease of the liver or the spleen rather than anxiety or depression. In spite of strenuous efforts within the general field of mental health, the 'Victorian whispers' of guilt and failure seem still to be firmly attached to many who are suffering from emotional or mental illness. It is therefore refreshing, and occasionally therapeutically effective, to have a different model with which to analyse and evaluate mental illness.

Vital energy

The Chinese believed that the force behind biological functions occurring in any living tissue necessitated vital energy, or 'Qi'. It is interesting to note that almost all systems of medicine other than allopathy have, to a greater or lesser extent, applied this concept of biological energy in one form or another. The Chinese concept of 'Qi' is both complex and tortuous; it has both substantive and functional elements. The substantive or material form of 'Qi' is represented by normal body nutrients such as food or gaseous exchange. The non-substantive form is the real but elusive concept of a vital force and goes some way to explain why an otherwise healthy individual feels full of energy one day and drained and rather unproductive the next. Intuitively, the idea that health and disease may be affected by the body's vital energy (or 'Qi') seems plausible, but as yet we have no objective or scientific measure which can be applied to this phenomenon.

The idea of a vital force is a very difficult concept for the allopath to accept, primarily because we are currently unable to measure its activity. Nevertheless, it represents the central assumption of the traditional Chinese approach to health and disease. Within the concepts of traditional Chinese medicine, disease occurs because of an abnormal flow of vital energy and symptoms can be cured or palliated by selecting acupuncture points that will return the body's energy to normal.

Pathogenesis

Disease results when the body is weakened and unable to resist the onslaught of pathogens. In Chinese medicine the agents that cause disease are given the names of meteorological conditions: an infection (often associated with a fever) is called a disease of heat, and a chronically painful joint is usually a disease of cold. These pathogens allow diseases to be grouped according to their broad symptoms. The pathogen wind is an interesting idea— within the context of traditional Chinese medicine wind means a changeable symptom. Therefore the type of muscular ache that often occurs in association with a viral infection would be classed as invasion by wind. The idea that disease is due to physical conditions is an intuitive explanation for many common aches and pains. People often complain that they 'caught a chill when they got wet', or that their 'neck is stiff after having slept in a draught'. The traditional Chinese concept of a pathogen represents a formalisation of this approach.

A particular pathogen usually presents with a defined symptom complex. By using the information gained from the history of the disease, and the physical examination of the patient, it is often possible to make a clear diagnosis of the pathogen causing the disease. If the patient has a fever, then heat is one of the pathogens involved in the disease process. Once this diagnosis has been made, specific acupuncture points can be used to disperse the pathogen: when heat is present specific points can be used to reduce fever. Within the context of animal experiments executed by the Chinese, it would appear that acupuncture points do exist which seem to reduce body temperature.

If the pathogen cold is responsible for a particular disease process, then heat must be used to treat it. Moxa is the Chinese version of the heat lamp and, as discussed earlier, the Chinese burn the dried leaves of *Artemisia vulgaris* over the areas that require heat. Heat, or more specifically smouldering moxa, provides a local treatment for a variety of chronic muscular aches.

Other factors may also cause disease, such as worry or eating contaminated food. The *Nei Ching* states that excessive grief, anxiety and over-thinking will cause a tumour (cancer). This idea has been supported by some recent studies which suggest that if a woman has a breast removed for cancer, she will survive longer if she is of a happy and relaxed disposition. The traditional Chinese ideas about pathogens, both internal and external, would seem to have some degree of validity when analysed in an objective manner with the aid of modern scientific and epidemiological techniques.

Diagnosis

One of the most difficult skills for the practitioner of traditional Chinese medicine is to define the specific organ affected by any particular disease. As with all systems of medicine, a detailed history often gives a very clear indication as to the diagnosis. If the acupuncturist understands the functions ascribed to each organ by the Chinese, then this will provide an essential and irreplaceable starting point from which a diagnosis can be made.

As well as observing and palpating the diseased area of the body, the ancient Chinese also palpated the pulse. Pulse palpation was achieved by feeling the radial pulse at three positions on each wrist, and by noting the pulse characteristics at the superficial and deep sites at each of these. The superficial pulse can be palpated at approximately systolic pressure and the deep pulse at approximately diastolic pressure. There are therefore six pulses at each wrist, three superficial and three deep. There are 12 main organs in the Chinese medical system and each of these is represented by one of the pulses at one of the wrist positions. It is unclear how the system of pulse diagnosis came into existence, but it had been refined and classified in detail by 500 BC, This method of diagnosis allows the whole body to be assessed and it also defines the relative balance between each of the organs. In addition, pulse diagnosis is said to give a clear idea of the type of disease process and pathogen causing that disease in any individual patient.

It is almost unbelievable to think that different organs can be represented by slight differences in the characteristics of the pulse in the right and left hands. The Chinese were not concerned with the rate or rhythm of the pulse, but with its detailed characteristics. For instance, the pulse may be defined as 'Fu' or 'Ch'en'. A 'Fu' pulse is described as a superficial pulse, it is light and flowing like a piece of wood floating on water, whereas a 'Ch'en' pulse is a deep pulse, like a stone thrown into water. These graphic descriptions can be recorded with the aid of a small peizo-electric pressure sensor on each of the pulse positions, and they can be visualised by the use of a six-channel oscilloscope (Fig. 1.4). The techniques and interpretation of electronic pulsography were discovered and systematised by Drs Yoo and Paik in West Germany and the system and its interpretation have been described in detail by Dr Kenyon (1983). When using electronic pulsography, it would seem that the description of the pulse characteristics can be verified by the recordings obtained. For instance, a superficial pulse is indeed superficial in that there is an upper deflection of the pulse wave on the recording and very little downward motion of the pulse in that position.

It is difficult to know exactly how to interpret the information obtained from the pulsograph. This machine does seem to provide some objective, but circumstantial, evidence that suggests that the traditional Chinese pulses may be of some value.

Use of the 12 pulses takes many years to learn to a standard of competence which will allow the acupuncturist to make a clear diagnosis. Although there are some people, both in China and in the West, who are able to diagnose by the use of the 12 pulses,

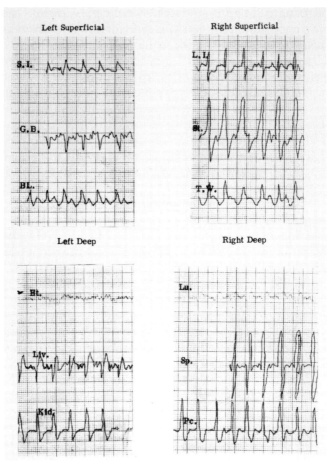

Fig. 1.4 A pulse recording.

they are few in number, and a modified system of diagnosis has therefore been developed by the Chinese. This allows a simple but relatively accurate system of traditional diagnosis to be taught and practised quite quickly and proficiently, the mainstays of this 'shorter method' being the use of a pulse generalisation and the tongue.

The pulse is not felt in any particular position but for its general character, hence the term 'pulse generalisation'. It can be felt at either wrist and classed as generally excessive or deficient, with perhaps ten intermediate categories. Other detailed diagnostic systems exist within traditional Chinese medicine, such as tongue diagnosis and diagnosis by smell etc. However, it would be inappropriate to discuss these techniques in detail in so short a chapter. This simpler method would appear to be almost as accurate as that involving the old traditional pulses and allows the acupuncturist to make an assessment of the five 'Zang' organs accurately, and after a fairly short period of training.

Point selection

The diagnosis of a particular problem does not tell the acupuncturist where to place a needle; a set of therapeutic rules must be applied to solve that problem. To a large degree, all medical systems are based on clinical experience, and acupuncture is no exception to this general rule.

The rules of point selection may be based on a wide range of approaches to acupuncture. The simplest, and most obvious, is the use of acupuncture in acute or chronic pain. In this instance, points may be selected purely by localising the most tender trigger zones and needling the tender points alone.

However, in many diseases, and in the case of pain, associated symptomatology may be present. This might include anxiety and/or depression or abdominal symptoms and indigestion which can sometimes be produced by analgesic or non-steroidal anti-inflammatory agents. In such instances it may be difficult, if not impossible, to select points purely based on the patient's localisation of pain. In disease processes such as asthma, where acupuncture has been shown to have a proven bronchodilator effect, point selection cannot be based on tender point localisation and does require some knowledge of traditional Chinese organ function and the empirical rules of point selection that exist within traditional Chinese medicine.

As already mentioned, there are particular points that can be used to disperse the invasion of specific pathogens such as heat or wind. The other rules of point selection are many and varied. For example, points can be selected on the basis of a law of five elements; this law assumes that each of the organs represents one of the five elements in traditional Chinese thought (earth, fire, water, metal and wood) and that they have a creating and destroying cycle. On each of the channels there are points representing one of these elements, and by applying a complex set of rules the diseased organ can be sedated (if it is overactive) or tonified (if it is underactive). There are also points on the back and front of the body that are said to represent specific organs, possibly through some as yet poorly defined viscerosomatic reflex. These too can be used to treat specific organs. There is a plethora of such rules, each of which can be applied in specific conditions and at specific times. Probably one of the biggest problems for any acupuncturist is to define the few points that will be most clinically effective in any particular condition. The skill of point selection (as with all skills in clinical medicine) is based largely on clinical experience; the rules of point selection give guidelines although they do not represent the complete answer for any particular problem.

Neurophysiological explanations for the mechanism of acupuncture and TENS

Acupuncture in the West is used mainly as a treatment for pain and is available in approximately three-quarters of the pain clinics in England and Wales. Consequently the vast majority of well-substantiated physiological theories that have been used to explain its mechanism centre around its effects on pain transmission and perception. Although we understand a great deal about the physiology and psychology of pain, no unified theory exists which can explain its mechanism, and there are many painful conditions whose pathophysiology is poorly documented. Therefore we cannot hope to provide a complete explanation for the apparent analgesic effects of acupuncture as we must accept that it is modifying a system that is only partially elucidated.

The gate control theory

It is probably sensible to think of the physiological changes initiated by both acupuncture and TENS as being mediated initially by the peripheral nervous system. The first theory that was used to explain acupuncture and TENS was the gate control theory developed by Melzack and Wall (1965). Pain seems to be carried by unmyelinated C fibres, and light touch by myelinated A fibres. The gate control theory states that these two inputs are integrated in the substantia gelatinosa (a structure in the dorsal horn of the spinal cord) and that onward transmission of pain is controlled by the balance of activity between the C and A fibres.

If C-fibre activity dominates, pain is perceived; A-fibre activity inhibits the central transmission (and subsequent perception) of pain.

Efforts to verify this theory experimentally have led to apparently conflicting conclusions. Direct electrostimulation of both the peripheral nerves and dorsal horn does result in analgesia. However, artificially stimulating A-fibre activity does not seem to abolish the pain produced by C-fibre stimulation. Acupuncture and TENS clearly activate (selectively) A-fibre activity (Nathan and Rudge, 1974). However, brief intense stimulation may cause prolonged pain relief, a phenomenon that is difficult to explain within the context of the gate control theory. Melzack has suggested that this phenomenon could be explained by either a 'central biasing mechanism', or by the abolition of proposed 'memory-like processes' through which pain may be mediated (Melzack, 1975).

The gate control theory implies that acupuncture and TENS should have their greatest effect if both C- and A-fibre activity occurs within the same dermatome. This does appear to be the case, but it is apparent that acupuncture can relieve pain on a bizarre heterosegmental basis, a phenomenon that cannot be explained solely by the gate control theory.

The thalamus, reticular activating system and descending inhibitory control

Melzack (1975) has suggested that because stimulation of the peri-aqueductal grey matter appears to diminish pain perception, some sort of central biasing mechanism may exist which apparently influences the transmission of painful stimuli in the neuraxis. More recent observations by Akil *et al.* (1976) and others have demonstrated that stimulation of both the peri-aqueductal grey and the nucleus raphe magnus results in analgesia that is probably endorphin mediated. It seems that neurons originating in these cerebral nuclei are capable of exerting important and potentially analgesic effects on the activity of the dorsal horn.

The reticular activating system also seems to influence pain perception; the analgesic effects of acupuncture in some instances seem to be unaffected by superficial cordotomy, but its effects are significantly influenced by the activity of the reticular activating system. This implies that the reticular activating system is possibly more important in certain specific situations than the dorsal horn in modifying pain perception and transmission (Chen-Yo *et al.*, 1975; Ke-Fi and Shu-Fang, 1977).

Chang (1973) has written extensively on the role of the thalamus in pain and how its functions may be altered by acupuncture. His animal studies indicate that the nuclei parafascicularis and centralis lateralis are essential for the integration of painful stimuli, and that their activity is influenced by acupuncture. Furthermore, this thalamic activity remains unaffected when the dorsal horn is destroyed, again suggesting that the reticular activating system is of vital importance in pain and may be a very major pathway for mediating the effects of acupuncture and TENS.

Viscerosomatic reflexes

For many years we have known that a wide variety of viscerosomatic reflexes exist, such as the scratch reflex in 'spinal' dogs. A large number of cutaneous stimuli appear to influence internal, often autonomic, functions; trigger points appear in angina and puncturing them with needles can alleviate cardiac pain. It is quite possible that many of the intersegmental effects of acupuncture could be explained by these reflexes and it is apparent that we understand very little about them. Acupuncture does appear to have an effect on a number of these viscerosomatic reflexes, but we have virtually no information about the exact mechanism through which cutaneous stimuli such as needle puncture can affect the autonomic nervous system (Mann, 1977). However, we can, with good reason, suppose that the autonomic nervous system is of vital importance in mediating many painful diseases, including chronic pain. Clearly this is a poorly defined area, but one which would benefit from further more detailed investigation.

Diffuse noxious inhibitory control

Evidence is available which demonstrates that any noxious stimuli (in rats) can modify pain perception by producing analgesia at distant sites in that animal (Le Bars *et al.*, 1979). Some authorities have suggested this represents acupuncture's mechanism of action. It may be that clumsy, painful or crude acupuncture techniques could be mediated through this pathway. Perhaps the effects of random needle puncture may produce analgesia through diffuse noxious inhibitory control. However, acupuncture and TENS are not usually painful and may have a prolonged and profound analgesic effect. Therefore diffuse noxious inhibitory control must be a mechanism which can only explain a small part of the complete picture.

Other neurological theories

Becker (1974) has suggested that acupuncture is mediated through a primitive nervous system. He has hypothesised that, as in many control systems involving high-energy processes, a control system involving signals of low energy could be present. He uses as support for this argument various detailed experiments on bone healing, leg regeneration in the salamander, and some detailed studies on the electrophysiological correlates of acupuncture points. However, whether the proposed transmission and control systems really exist, or can be modified by acupuncture, remains unproven.

Is there a neurological explanation?

Many of these neurological explanations may at first seem confusing. In some instances the same sets of observations seem to have been used to support rather different hypotheses. Furthermore, in most of the studies which have provided evidence for the mechanism of acupuncture, animal models have been used. It may be wrong to assume that information obtained from the study of noxious stimuli in animals (often decerebrate animals) can be used to explain the neurological implications of inserting an acupuncture needle into man for the treatment of chronic pain. Many neurophysiologists do not consider acute experimental pain, even in human volunteers, to be necessarily working through the same mechanism as chronic pain. In spite of these criticisms, acupuncture and TENS do seem to be having an effect at many sites in the central nervous system. It is probable that a complex series of feedback loops operates at segmental, intersegmental, medullary, midbrain and thalamic levels. It is likely that each of the theories discussed represents part of the truth rather than the complete explanation of all the observed phenomena.

Endorphins

It has been recognised for some years that morphine and other opiates are excellent and powerful analgesics. Recently, naturally occurring opiates (endorphins and enkephalins) have been isolated (Hughes *et al.*, 1975). Enkephalins were first discovered in porcine brain. There are two types, leu- and met-enkephalin, both are pentapeptides. The endorphins are composed of 30 amino acids, and are found in the serum and in cerebrospinal fluid as well as in a wide variety of sites in the central nervous system, including the spinal cord and in particular the dorsal horn (Dupont *et al.*, 1980).

A large number of studies both on man and in a variety of animal models have demonstrated that electro-acupuncture and TENS promote the release of these chemicals into the cerebrospinal fluid and peri-aqueductal grey. Sjolund *et al.* (1977) have demonstrated that acupuncture causes the release of endorphins in a segmental manner. If points on the distribution of the cervical dermatomes are stimulated, then endorphins appear to be released in the cervical region of the cord, not in the lumbar region. Pomeranz (1981) has produced a vast number of excellent studies evaluating the effects of acupuncture with respect to the possibility that it might be mediated through endorphins; most of this work has been on mice. It would appear from these studies that there is excellent and persuasive evidence largely supporting the acupuncture–endorphin hypothesis.

In 1975 a Chinese neurosurgeon, Dr Wen, reported that symptoms of heroin withdrawal could be alleviated by electro-acupuncture. This resulted in a collaborative study with Professor Besser's unit at St Bartholomew's Hospital (London) in which it was shown that electro-acupuncture caused a significant rise of met-enkephalin in the cerebrospinal fluid of such addicts. Electro-acupuncture in patients with chronic pain showed an increase in cerebrospinal fluid levels of β-endorphin, but met-enkephalin levels were unchanged in these patients. These results suggest that the mechanisms involved in heroin withdrawal and pain relief may be different, although both appear to be mediated by naturally occurring opiates (Clement-Jones *et al.*, 1979):

Having established that endorphin release can be stimulated by acupuncture, it is necessary to demonstrate that these physiological changes do correlate with clinical pain relief. Electrical stimulation of the periventricular brain in man causes profound analgesia accompanied by a massive increase in β-endorphin levels, and intrathecal administration of β-endorphin produces a long-lasting analgesic effect in cancer patients. It has also been noted that patients with chronic pain seem to have a low level of β-endorphin in their cerebrospinal fluid, but that these levels do not seem to correlate with the severity or duration of pain. A similar case has been made for the mechanism of TENS, in that it has also been shown that this form of stimulation therapy causes a rise in β-endorphin levels within the cerebrospinal fluid.

Naloxone, a morphine antagonist, does largely reverse the effects of exogenous opiates such as morphine, and should by implication reverse any endorphin-based effects such as the analgesia created by acupuncture. The weight of evidence available shows that acupuncture is probably *not* reversed by naloxone (Chapman *et al.*, 1983). This may be because naloxone, although it displaces opium and morphine from their receptor sites, does not displace endorphins. Or as Chapman *et al.* (1983) believe, it may be one of several important 'chinks' in their widely accepted acupuncture–endorphin hypothesis. Chapman *et al.* have provided very persuasive arguments that suggest fluctuations in endorphin levels are incidental rather than central in mediating the effects of acupuncture and TENS.

Effects on other neurotransmitters

Acupuncture has apparently wide-ranging and well-documented effects on a number of important neurotransmitters, and these are excellently reviewed by Jisheng (1979). It is known to cause a significant increase in 5-HT (serotonin) in rat brain, and other studies have revealed that both the synthesis and utilisation of central 5-HT are accelerated during acupuncture. Furthermore, double-blind studies on the effects of acupuncture anaesthesia for dental extraction show that acupuncture was significantly strengthened by the prior oral administration of clomipramine, which blocks the re-uptake of 5-HT, thus raising its functional activity.

Acetylcholine also has an effect on acupuncture analgesia: blockade of acetylcholine synthesis by intravenous injection of hemicholine (in rats) impedes the effect of acupuncture analgesia. The effect of acupuncture analgesia in both rabbits and rats could be partially blocked by atropine and potentiated by eserine.

Dopamine agonists such as apomorphine increase the effect of acupuncture analgesia, while administration of droperidol (a dopamine antagonist) decreases its effect. Intravenous injection of the chemical precursors of norepinephrine partially blocks the effect of acupuncture analgesia, and the administration of an agonist (clonidine) of the central α-receptors also depresses the analgesic effect that can be obtained from acupuncture on rats. Phentolamine (an α-receptor antagonist) has been found to augment the effect of acupuncture analgesia. It therefore seems likely that dopamine (through dopamine receptors) and noradrenaline (through α-receptors) exert antagonist effects on acupuncture analgesia.

Propranolol causes a decrease in the effect of acupuncture analgesia in rats, which is in line with the clinical finding that propranolol makes acupuncture anaesthesia in man less effective. This suggests a facilitating effect of α-receptors occurs during the process. Acupuncture has also been shown to lower the cerebral noradrenaline content, apparently as a result of greater utilisation and synthesis of this chemical.

These arguments strongly support the notion that acupuncture has a fundamental effect on many central neurotransmitters.

Psychological mechanisms

Although the majority of mechanisms suggested for acupuncture have concentrated on physiological theories, some more psychological explanations are available. There has been some suggestion that particular types of patients respond to acupuncture, often the suggestible and anxious. Studies which have analysed personality types and correlated these with response to treatment do not provide a clear-cut result; it is currently impossible to predict which patients will respond to this therapy.

Hypnosis

Early reports of acupuncture seemed incredible, particularly from those who visited China during the late 1960s and early 1970s and observed acupuncture analgesia. Many authoritative voices proposed, in all seriousness, that acupuncture was in effect working through hypnotic suggestibility. Superficially there seemed to be many similarities between acupuncture analgesia and hypnotic states. However, it has been shown by several authors that the patients' potential for hypnotic suggestibility in no way correlates with their response to acupuncture. Furthermore, acupuncture analgesia, for a particular limb, overcomes the hypnotic suggestion that that limb is hypersensitive. While the exact mechanism of hypnosis remains unclear, the evidence available to date implies that these two therapies are probably working through largely different mechanisms (Pomeranz and Chiu, 1976).

The placebo effect

Acupuncture is a dramatic, and in lay terms, mystical therapy, and therefore almost certainly has some element of suggestion within it. However, if acupuncture were purely a placebo, then physical placebos similar to it should result in a higher placebo effect than that noted from placebo medication. As will be demonstrated in my discussion of clinical trials, physical placebos display the same degree of efficacy as that expected from placebo medication. Therefore acupuncture is having a far greater effect than that expected from a placebo alone.

Any therapy, particularly for painful conditions, is more likely to be of value if the relationship between the doctor and patient is effective in reducing anxiety. Acupuncture is frequently practised (in the United Kingdom) in the setting of a private clinic where the patient receives both time and sympathy from the doctor. Consequently some of the success claimed by acupuncture could be attributed to the relationship between the therapist and the patient rather than to the therapy itself. The extent of this factor remains undefined, and even though it is a phenomenon that is difficult to investigate objectively, it is most unlikely that it represents the complete explanation for the efficacy of this therapy.

Race

Early reports of acupuncture in China have implied that this was a useful therapy for the Chinese but it would never work in the West. Perhaps this was because the inscrutable face of the Orient was thought to be almost resistant to pain. Studies on pain and personality have shown that Orientals are at least as susceptible to experimental pain as Occidental races, in fact there is some suggestion that Orientals have a significantly lower pain tolerance than Caucasians. It therefore seems unlikely that race has any significant effect on the outcome from this form of therapy (Chapman *et al.*, 1982).

The mechanism of acupuncture in the treatment of non-painful conditions

Acupuncture has been used as a therapy for many non-painful conditions, and a clear effect from acupuncture has been reported on the immune system, the gall bladder, the smooth muscle of the bronchial tree and the coronary arteries, to name but a few (*National Symposium of Acupuncture Moxibustion and Acupuncture Anaesthesia, 1979*). Acupuncture has also been shown to cause a number of fundamental changes in the autonomic system and several experiments attest to its influence on the gastrointestinal tract. These studies demonstrate that needle puncture is having a fundamental effect on aspects of the nervous system that control internal functions rather than just pain, and the observations represent just a small part of a growing body of literature that describes the actions of acupuncture in non-painful conditions.

However, such changes have been poorly researched and their mechanism is unclear. Furthermore, very few clinical trials have been published which have attempted to evaluate the symptomatic or curative effects of acupuncture on non-painful conditions. Consequently we know very little about the mechanism and the clinical effects of acupuncture in such situations, although it is very likely that many such effects are mediated through the autonomic nervous system.

Conclusion

As with almost all therapies, there is no definitive answer as to exactly how acupuncture works, either for pain or for the treatment of non-painful conditions. However, there are a large number of exceptionally well documented observations which lead us to suppose that acupuncture is having a fundamental effect on our physiological functions, an effect which does apparently modify the transmission and perception of pain. From the evidence available it would take a very brave and possibly slightly headstrong person to suggest that acupuncture is having its effects simply because it is a dramatic form of therapy.

Unfortunately, the information available from these detailed neurophysiological studies does not provide the practising acupuncturist with enough detail to allow him to select needling sites for specific problems. Therefore, in spite of the wealth of physiological evidence that has become available over the last decade, the practising acupuncturist must largely be dependent on empirical information gleaned from traditional Chinese texts if he is to be effective in treating patients.

Acupuncture, the patient's view

A number of people are frightened by the thought of acupuncture as 'needles' or injections strike an unpleasant chord in our memories. Body acupuncture is not a particularly painful experience in skilled hands. It is much less traumatic than an injection as it involves the use of a small-diameter atraumatic needle with a dowled, and not a cutting, point. Consequently tissue damage, bruising and bleeding are far less likely to occur with acupuncture than with an injection. Most acupuncturists will insert between 8 and 12 needles in any acupuncture session.

Needling sensation

The Chinese believe that if acupuncture is to obtain its maximum effect, it is necessary for the acupuncturist to obtain needling sensation over each acupuncture point used. This involves the needle being moved slightly (and relatively painlessly) while it is in the skin. The sensation experienced by the patient is largely subjective and may be quite variable. Needling sensation is not painful, but it is a dull, bursting or numb feeling around the site of the inserted needle. Occasionally sensations may travel up and down the channel on which the acupuncture point is situated; for instance, the stimulation of an acupuncture point on the right knee may precipitate a strange burning or numb sensation in the right ankle. Needling sensation is probably best defined by the statement: 'When needling sensation is experienced the needle no longer feels like a needle!' Some acupuncturists use electrostimulation, and when doing so, the stimulator should be adjusted to cause a pleasant tingling sensation over the acupuncture points being stimulated. Many Western doctors, particularly anaesthetists, believe that acupuncture is synonymous with such stimulation therapy. The Chinese believe that the use of electrostimulation does not replace the need to obtain needling sensation, and that it is important but limited in its uses. The real treatment advantages of manual stimulation of the needle, versus simple needle puncture, versus electro-acupuncture, have not really been adequately tested. However, there is some circumstantial evidence that suggests needling sensation elicits neurophysiological changes which do not occur in response to simple needle puncture. In my opinion the routine use of electrostimulation probably adds very little to the efficacy of treatment, and in some cases may actually be counterproductive. I would support the Chinese view of the use of electrostimulation and suggest that its main value is in the treatment of nerve injury (such as in a stroke), as an aid to providing prolonged analgesia (such as that required during labour and delivery or other operative procedures), and as a method for promoting endorphin release in the treatment of addictions.

Will I get better?

Probably the most common thought in patients' minds is the desire to know whether acupuncture is going to solve their problem. As with almost all medical treatments, it is impossible to predict with certainty the outcome at the onset of treatment. Acupuncture is no exception to this rule, although certainly for pain the information available would suggest that this form of therapy is at least as effective as conventional treatments and certainly more effective than the placebo. In non-painful conditions the situation is far from clear.

The majority of the acupuncture practised in the United Kingdom is within the private sphere. There is considerable evidence to suggest that patients who pay for therapy are more likely to obtain therapeutic benefit from that treatment. This necessarily enhances the effect that can be obtained by acupuncture (this applies to the practice of *all* medicine in the private sector). The studies quoted describing the effect of acupuncture in chronic pain have reported its therapeutic effects in non-fee-paying, carefully selected groups of patients. It is probable that the effect of acupuncture in normal clinical practice is greater than 60%. I do not wish to imply that I believe acupuncture should remain in the private sector, particularly as within our teaching programme at the centre we have devoted a considerable amount of time and effort to promoting the practice of acupuncture within the National Health Service. However, it is important that the prudent and objective practitioner recognises the many and varied factors that comprise an effective therapeutic result, and necessarily the environment in which the therapy is practised is one of these factors.

Response to treatment

It is almost impossible to predict how a patient will respond to acupuncture. Very occasionally, one treatment is all that is required, whereas other people may need a number of treatments to gain the same result for the same disease. In general most people, and their problems, do not respond magically to one treatment, and between four and eight treatment sessions may be required in order to obtain the best results from acupuncture.

Acupuncture usually works in stages. The first two or three treatments represent a process of 'understanding the needs of the patient', and are therefore a sort of experiment designed to assess the specific requirements for that person in that particular condition. Some people respond to classical Chinese body acupuncture, whereas others respond better to ear acupuncture. This partially reflects the skill of the acupuncturist in the use of specific techniques, but it also represents the fact that the body responds in a slightly different way to different stimuli. A patient may respond to a particular approach for a specific condition and then stop improving halfway through the treatment, necessitating the use of an alternative approach.

If patients experience some symptomatic improvement at the first consultation, then they often gain considerable relief from a course of acupuncture. Equally, many people who do not obtain symptomatic improvement at the first consultation may also gain a great deal from acupuncture. However it is a good prognostic sign if there is some instant improvement, although this rarely lasts for more than a day or two and may last only a few minutes. Each subsequent treatment should give a better and more prolonged result, and symptoms should gradually begin to disappear as treatment becomes effective.

Three or four treatments should be adequate to assess

whether a patient will respond to acupuncture. If there has been no response to treatment after the first three sessions, then it is doubtful whether any response will occur. This should be taken as a general guideline and not as an unbreakable rule, as sometimes the symptoms of a particular condition may be fluctuant and it may be difficult to obtain a clear assessment of the results of treatment. Occasionally the patient may find it difficult to remember exactly what the condition was like three weeks before, so it is wise for him to keep a diary and assess day by day changes that are occurring in the problem being treated.

Most acupuncturists will continue to treat patients until there is no further improvement in their condition. The response tends to level off towards the end of treatment (usually after about five to eight treatments) and this signifies that further treatment will probably not give further benefit. Acupuncturists in the West tend to treat people on a weekly basis; in China treatment is given daily but this seems to be more from habit than for any good medical reason. Weekly treatments allow both the patient and the acupuncturist to gain a clear assessment of the progress and response to therapy.

If acupuncture is used as a treatment for pain, then it is nearly always of a palliative nature. The Chinese claim, in some instances, that acupuncture can have a curative effect in the treatment of conditions such as acute infections; this claim requires further substantive proof. The traditional Chinese approach is to attempt to maintain the patient in a state of health, and regular three-monthly treatment patterns may therefore be justified. However, most acupuncturists feel it is better and more ethically justifiable to treat patients when symptoms recur. If the condition is self-limiting, such as an acute sprain, then obviously no further treatment is required after normal pain-free function has returned.

Sometimes the patient may experience a temporary worsening of symptoms due to acupuncture; this is a response to treatment and in general is a good sign, usually only lasting for a day or two and being followed by improvement. Similar reactions may occur in the use of all of the alternative therapies, although they are not commonly met with by those prescribing allopathic treatment.

Some patients are very sensitive to acupuncture and may respond to normal needle stimulation by over-reacting. If a reaction occurs, the patient should be stimulated less at the next treatment session, this usually means giving a shorter and less aggressive treatment. Sometimes improvement may be very delayed and symptoms may not clear until the treatment has ceased. Occasionally patients who have been abandoned, with no improvement after three weeks, will suddenly find improvement some weeks after the cessation of acupuncture.

Although I have attempted to outline general guidelines, as with all clinical disciplines the general rules are not always obeyed. Nevertheless, it is important for those interested in acupuncture, or wishing to refer patients to acupuncturists, to have a clear idea of the likely response to treatment. In many instances the patients will ask the referring doctor or physiotherapist about the progress of their treatment and it is helpful to the therapist and reassuring for the patient to have some knowledge about the likely response to therapy.

The clinical effects of acupuncture therapy

Acupuncture has been used by the Chinese for at least the last two millennia. In most instances it was used to treat minor ailments, acute infections and as a prophylactic measure against disease. The rich Chinese patient was seen regularly and treated so that he could remain in a state of good health. In the West, acupuncture has been suggested as a therapy for a wide range of conditions, most of them chronic. In many instances it has been used after the Western therapy has failed to produce therapeutic benefit. Consequently a treatment initially designed and conceived as a system of primary care is currently being tested as a system of secondary or in some cases tertiary care.

It is indeed surprising that this therapy is surviving such a stringent test. As with our understanding of the proposed physiological mechanisms of acupuncture, the majority of information available about its clinical effectiveness centres around its use in chronic painful conditions. Rather than present a morass of unsubstantiated, descriptive clinical impressions, I have chosen to concentrate on the clinical trials that have made some attempt to provide a realistic assessment of acupuncture's therapeutic efficacy.

Painful conditions

Unfortunately, much of our current knowledge about the

clinical effects of acupuncture has been based on descriptive studies, which claim that acupuncture is effective in treating almost all types of chronic pain. An extensive literature search has revealed 20 controlled clinical trials that have attempted to evaluate acupuncture as a treatment for painful, mainly musculoskeletal, conditions. These studies can be divided into three broad categories: acupuncture as compared with conventional therapy, acupuncture as compared with random insertion of acupuncture needles, and acupuncture compared with a physical placebo.

Acupuncture versus conventional therapy

Six studies have been published in which the efficacy of acupuncture is compared with conventional therapy for musculoskeletal pain; the results obtained are summarised in Table 1.1. All these studies are simple, comparative exercises involving carefully specified groups of patients with the same musculoskeletal condition, none involves cross-over or 'blind' therapy.

In some of the projects very few patients were entered; for instance, Man and Baragar studied 20 patients with rheumatoid arthritis affecting the knee, 10 in each group, and Fernandes *et al.* used 5 treatment regimens for shoulder pain, with 12 patients in each treatment group. Consequently the results and subsequent conclusions that emerge from such limited research must be interpreted with caution. The highly successful results claimed by Man and Baragar should be balanced against the more depressing conclusion of Fernandes *et al.*, the truth probably existing between the two extremes.

Size is not the only obstacle that impedes a clear interpretation of these studies. Gunn *et al.* reported a trial in which acupuncture was added to a conventional treatment regimen for chronic low back pain; 56 patients were entered into the study, all of whom failed to benefit from 8 weeks' conventional therapy; 27 continued with conventional therapy, while 29 received acupuncture and conventional therapy. The acupuncture group obtained a significantly better treatment result with respect to pain relief than those continuing their conventional therapy. It is difficult to accept that a group of patients receiving a failed treatment regimen can realistically be thought of as a control group compared with patients being offered a new extra treatment such as acupuncture.

Table 1.1 Acupuncture compared with other physical therapies. (Success at the end of treatment expressed as a percentage of patients entered into each treatment group.)

References	Drugs (NSAID) and steroid injections	Acu- puncture	Physio- therapy	Problem
1. Junnila (1982)	32	61		Osteoarthritis of large joints
2. Fernandes *et al.* (1980)	50	50	50	Shoulder pain
3. Milligan *et al.* (1980)		82	48	Osteoarthritis of knees
4. Man and Baragar (1974)	10	90		Rheumatoid arthritis of knees
5. Gunn *et al.* (1980)		62	15	Low back pain
6. Brattenberg (1983)	30	68		Tennis elbow

The average response to drugs is 30%. The average response to acupuncture is 68%. The average response to physiotherapy is 38%.

1. *American Journal of Acupuncture*; 10:241–346. 2. *Lancet*; 1:208–09. 3. From paper presented at Fifteenth International Congress on Rheumatology, Paris. 4. *Journal of Rheumatology*; 1:126–9. 5. *Spine*; 5:279–91. 6. *Pain*; 16:285–8.

Nevertheless, acupuncture does emerge as a consistently better analgesic therapy than other treatments for the conditions being studied. Junnila makes the comment that not only is acupuncture better than a non-steroidal anti-inflammatory agent (Feldene) for osteoarthritis pain, but it is also virtually free from side-effects.

Acupuncture versus random insertion of acupuncture needles

Ten studies have been published using the model of random needling versus acupuncture. These studies have assumed that the therapeutic benefits obtained from the random needling are purely the result of a placebo effect, thus implying that needling in an inappropriate area of the body for the disease being treated does not produce a physiological change in the transmission and perception of pain. Such an assumption is probably incorrect as physiological evidence is available which suggests that any noxious stimulus can attenuate pain elsewhere in the body through the mechanism of diffuse noxious inhibitory control. Therefore, studies using random needling are probably best thought of as an evaluation of acupuncture versus a less effective form of needle puncture. Table 1.2 summarises the results obtained.

Table 1.2   Acupuncture compared with random needling. (Success at the end of treatment expressed as a percentage of patients entered.)

References	Random needling	Acupuncture	Problem
1. Moore and Berk (1976)	39	23	Shoulder pain
2. Hansen *et al.* (1981)	45	75	Facial pain
3. Co *et al.* (1979)	50	81	Pain from sickling crisis
4. Matsumoto *et al.* (1974)	Only mean scores given		Shoulder pain
5. Gaw *et al.* (1975)	36	58	Osteoarthritis pain
6. Godfrey and Morgan (1978)	54	63	Musculoskeletal pain
7. Weintraub *et al.* (1975)	Only mean scores given		Musculoskeletal pain
8. Lee *et al.* (1975)	—	70	Chronic pain
9. Mendelson *et al.* (1983)	22	26 (mean scores)	Back pain
10. Edelist *et al.* (1976)	40	46	Back pain

The average effect obtained from random needling is 41%. The average effect obtained from acupuncture is 55%.

1. *American Internal Medicine*; **84**:381–4. 2. *Acta Neurochirurgica*; **59**:279. 3. *Pain*; **7**:181–5. 4. *American Surgery*; **40**:200–05. 5 *New England Journal of Medicine*; **293**:375–8. 6. *Journal of Rheumatology*; **5**:121–4. 7. *Clinical and Pharmacological Therapy*; **17**:248. 8. *Journal of the American Medical Association*; **232**:1133–5. 9. *American Journal of Medicine*; **74**:49–55. 10. *Canadian Anaesthesiology Society Journal*; **23**:303–06.

The effectiveness claimed for both acupuncture and random needling does not seem to be altered by the study method chosen. Some of these studies involved the use of cross-over design, while others compared the effects of acupuncture with those of random needling. In all the studies the patients were unaware as to whether they were receiving acupuncture or random needling, and in one study the acupuncturist himself was not aware of which therapy he was administering!

Most of these studies involved musculoskeletal pain, and in spite of different trial designs and definitions of success or failure, the overall response to acupuncture is similar to that demonstrated in Table 1.1.

Previously published data suggest that a physical placebo should result in 30% of patients experiencing significant pain relief, random needling in a 50% response, and acupuncture in a 70% response (Lewith and Machin, 1983). The average response rates obtained in the studies comparing acupuncture and random needling are in broad agreement with this predicted response. The majority of these studies cannot individually be expected to produce a statistically significant result (at the $P = 0.05$ level) as only small numbers of patients have been entered into each clinical trial. However, the overall reported success of acupuncture is greater than that from random needling.

Acupuncture versus placebo

Two studies have been published using placebo acupuncture. In Junnila's study (1982) patients who could be treated lying face down were entered and the placebo involved pinching the back near to the site of needle insertion. Jensen *et al.* (1979) superficially pricked the skin over the acupuncture point that should have received treatment. It could be argued that both these placebos are really more like random needling than a true placebo. Two trials have been published in which another physical placebo has been compared with acupuncture. MacDonald *et al.* (1983) compared acupuncture with a large defunctioned eight-channel obstetric monitor. The machine, when switched on, produced both audio and visual signals (flashing lights); patients were connected to this equipment via surface electrodes on their back, with a wire from the surface electrodes to the machine. No known stimulus was transferred from the machine to the patients. Lewith *et al.* (1983) studied post-herpetic neuralgia, randomly allocating patients to placebo and acupuncture groups. A defunctioned transcutaneous nerve stimulator was used to provide the placebo.

The results obtained from these four studies are summarised in Table 1.3. It has been previously shown that a defunctioned TENS machine, i.e. a physical placebo, will produce a placebo response of the order of 30%. These four clinical trials all noted a placebo response of this magnitude, a reaction similar to that expected from placebo medication. The response to acupuncture was broadly in agreement with that noted in studies comparing acupuncture with other physical treatments and with random needling—that is, approximately 60% (see Tables 1.1 and 1.2).

Table 1.3 Acupuncture compared with placebo. (Success at the end of treatment expressed as a percentage of patients entered in each treatment group.)

References	Placebo	Acupuncture	Problem
1. Junnila (1982)	22	72	Musculoskeletal pain
2. Jensen *et al.* (1979)	50	68	Headache
3. MacDonald *et al.* (1983)	25	75	Back pain
4. Lewith *et al.* (1983)	21	24	Post-herpetic neuralgia

The average placebo response is 30%. The average acupuncture resonse is 60%.

1. *American Journal of Acupuncture*; 10:259–62. 2. *Scandinavian Journal of Dental Research*; 87:373–80. 3. *Annals of the Royal College of Surgeons*; 65:44–6. 4. *Pain*; 17:361–8.

Conclusion

Many of the studies involve small numbers of patients and some trials have been poorly designed with an unclear definition of the success or failure of the therapy. Although in the statistical sense it is incorrect to analyse results as averages (see Tables 1.1, 1.2 and 1.3), such an approach does provide a simple system for balancing the enthusiast against the pessimist and thereby, it is hoped, producing a realistic view of the effects of acupuncture on chronic pain. There is obviously a real need for further clinical studies based on the clinical and physiological evidence available. Lewith and Machin (1983) have suggested clinical and statistical methods for future research designed to evaluate the effects of acupuncture in painful conditions.

The results quoted in Tables 1.1, 1.2 and 1.3 refer to the effects of treatment at the end of the course of therapy. Acupuncture, like many analgesics, works for a limited period of time. Milligan *et al.* (1980) found its analgesic effects to have completely disappeared after approximately 6 months, whereas Brattenberg (1983) reported that approximately 60% of her patients remained either pain free or very much better at 6 months' follow-up. In nine of the studies quoted no follow-up was included, therefore it is difficult to assess clearly the long-term effects of acupuncture. All the studies that include a follow-up period demonstrate that the effect of acupuncture does diminish with time, thereby implying the patient will need further therapy directed at providing analgesia.

However, the information available allows us to deduce the following conclusions for the conditions studied.

1. Acupuncture has a significant effect in approximately 60% of patients suffering from chronic pain.

2. This effect is greater than that of a placebo and probably greater than that of random needling.

3. Acupuncture therapy is as effective as other conventional treatments for pain, such as physiotherapy and drugs, and is likely to cause fewer reactions than analgesics and anti-inflammatory medications.

Non-painful conditions

Addictions

Claims have been made that acupuncture is of value in alleviating the withdrawal symptoms that occur in a wide variety of addictions. These include addiction to hard drugs such as heroin and morphine, foods (obesity) and cigarettes. As acupuncture can artificially increase the release of endogenous opiates, it is almost certainly going to be of assistance in alleviating withdrawals in hard-drug addiction; however, clinical trials to prove this effect are currently unavailable. It is possible that tobacco addiction may in some way be endorphin mediated, although this hypothesis remains largely unproven. Nevertheless, smokers clearly experience severe withdrawal symptoms. Clinical trials are available which suggest that acupuncture is a good method for helping people to stop smoking, resulting in approximately 20% of patients studied abstaining totally from cigarette consumption 6 months after treatment has ceased. This figure summarises the information available from a good number of clinical trials and represents a conservative evaluation of the results claimed by some authors.

Treatment of so-called food addiction or obesity with acupuncture alone has a far from proven efficacy. Many acupuncturists seeing obese patients are in private practice and they are not only offering acupuncture, but usually some sort of diet associated with regular consultations and repeated weight recordings. Patients often lose weight in such therapeutic environments and this may well be partially due to acupuncture. However, more detailed studies are required before such assumptions can be proven.

Internal diseases

The Chinese, as well as a number of European authorities, have made many claims about the positive benefits of acupuncture in a broad range of internal diseases such as colitis, asthma, anxiety and depression, peptic ulcers, and as a general boost to the immune system and treatment of infectious diseases. The well-documented effects of acupuncture on the autonomic nervous system and central neurotransmission make it quite possible to envisage a variety of mechanisms through which such effects could be achieved. However, no definite mechanisms have emerged which appear to explain the effects of acupuncture in non-painful conditions.

Furthermore, few good clinical trials exist in this area and so many of the claims as to the real therapeutic benefit provided by acupuncture in the treatment of internal disease remain largely untested. It is essential to retain an open mind about its potential; above all else acupuncture is a safe therapy and, if used responsibly, in many instances may be preferable to a conventional treatment of equivalent therapeutic efficacy but with more side-effects. Accepted wisdom is often an irresistible force in medicine. It is a brave GP who does not prescribe antibiotics for a sore, red ear, but in spite of such 'tribal customs' there is little real evidence that antibiotics do much good and a growing body of information indicating that the indiscriminate use of antibiotics may be harmful. Acupuncture may prove to be of real value in the treatment of some internal diseases and its therapeutic benefits should not be dismissed lightly, particularly in view of the inadequacy of many allopathic therapies.

Can we assess the effects of acupuncture?

It is apparent, from the lack of detailed information about the clinical effects of acupuncture, particularly as a treatment for non-painful conditions, that much more information is required before a balanced judgement can be reached. The central difficulty in substantiating its effects is associated with the need to design and subsequently effect more thorough studies; the major problem being that acupuncture is not a therapy that can readily be tested within the conventional double-blind cross-over study. The information available suggests that acupuncture retains its effects for a limited period of time (for instance 6 months in arthritic problems of the knee), but unfortunately this temporal effect is unpredictable. In some instances, effects such as analgesia may be present for an hour or two, and for other patients receiving exactly the same treatment, 1 or 2 years of almost complete pain relief can occur. Sometimes there is immediate improvement in symptomatology and sometimes improvement is slowly progressive, its major effects becoming apparent after the treatment has ceased. These observations are common for many physical treatments. Therefore designing a study which includes cross-over makes it almost impossible to interpret the results with clarity; consequently studies must be designed on a comparative basis.

Comparative studies require a control group and although it would be perfectly legitimate to compare acupuncture with conventional treatments, it is also necessary to compare it with a physical placebo in order to obtain a clear evaluation of its real effect. As mentioned earlier, random needling is probably a very poor system for providing a control group with which to compare acupuncture. It is possible to conceive of a physical placebo, for instance a defunctioned transcutaneous nerve stimulator (mock TENS) will produce a placebo response of the order of 30%.

If a study were to compare acupuncture with mock TENS, it

could be argued that different therapists should provide the two different treatments. If this occurred there would be a danger of comparing the enthusiasm of the therapist rather than the treatments. If the same therapist provides both treatments, then one particular treatment may be 'sold' in a less than enthusiastic manner to the patients. One of these options must be chosen, but both have faults. Within the context of acupuncture trials it is difficult to conceive of a valid placebo which can be used consistently without the therapist's knowledge.

The measurement of a subjective phenomenon such as chronic pain, anxiety or breathlessness has proved difficult. However, some simple and apparently reasonably effective methods are available which can be used to measure treatment outcome for some of these symptoms. Prior to the inception of any study, clear definitions of the success or failure of therapy must be integrated into the system for measuring outcome.

The most common problem with the clinical trials published to date is that too few patients have been entered into the studies to allow a statistically significant result to emerge. If a significant result has been obtained, then its validity is often questionable because of the potential risk of a Type II error when interpreting the results. Trial size can safely be reduced by comparing two widely different treatments such as acupuncture (with a predicted 60% response rate) versus a physical placebo (with a predicted 30% response rate). As many symptoms tend to return when using acupuncture, survival curve analysis rather than a comparative statistical test would be a more appropriate method. Survival curve analysis can be used safely with slightly smaller treatment groups. A complete review of the relevant statistical methods for studies designed to evaluate the effects of acupuncture has been published previously (Lewith and Machin, 1983).

Some studies have evaluated the effects of acupuncture without making any realistic attempts to analyse separately the natural history of the different types of conditions within the trial. Ideally, a single disease should be studied and the entry criteria should be designed to define a relatively homogeneous group of patients.

In summary, acceptable studies designed to evaluate the effects of acupuncture should be single-blind comparative trials, initially using a physical placebo and perhaps later comparing the effects of acupuncture with more conventional therapies. If acupuncture is to become an 'accepted' therapy, studies based on these principles are mandatory.

Adverse reactions that can be caused by acupuncture

Probably the most important common and potentially dangerous adverse reaction that may result from the insertion of an acupuncture needle is the transmission of serum hepatitis. Acupuncture needles are like any other reusable piece of surgical equipment and must be properly cleaned and sterilised before they are used on patients. This procedure is simple and can be achieved by high temperatures alone, by steam sterilisation under pressure (autoclaving) or the use of commercially available chemical sterilisers such as Cidex. These precautions should always be followed with any piece of equipment that may be in contact with blood, blood products or any of the body's mucosal surfaces. Therefore, with a modicum of medical common sense, serum hepatitis should not present a risk to the competent practitioner.

If needles are inserted too deeply into the chest wall, particularly over the upper part of the thoracic spine, then they may penetrate through the muscle and into the pleura. Any competent practitioner of acupuncture will be well aware of this potential hazard and there are fairly simple procedures which need to be followed in order to avoid this possibility. Therefore a knowledge of simple anatomy, i.e. the position of the lungs, combined with adherence to a few simple clinical rules will overcome the potential risk of a pneumothorax occurring.

As already mentioned, some patients become a little worse after the first or perhaps the second acupuncture treatment. Acupuncturists usually call this a 'reaction', and more often than not it signifies that the patient will improve. Such reactions usually only occur for 24, or at the most 48, hours and represent a response to treatment. If a patient has a reaction, the acupuncturist would be well advised to use fewer needles, leaving them in situ for a shorter period of time so that a similar situation does not occur after subsequent therapy.

Many people, when learning acupuncture, are very worried about the fact that acupuncture needles may penetrate nerves or small blood vessels. Occasionally a small amount of bleeding at the site of needle insertion does occur, and if a rather friable vein wall is needled, then a small local bruise can result. These are not dangerous adverse reactions, and judging by the information available from the literature and from my own clinical experience, such events have never been reported as serious adverse reactions. Local infection at the site of needle insertion is also almost unheard of, even though needles are inserted into unsterilised skin. The needle is of small diameter and has a dowelled rather than cutting edge. Consequently it is less likely to introduce infection than a hypodermic needle which actively 'cores' out a small cylinder of skin and, by implication, injects bacteria and superficial tissue into the deeper tissue layers.

Faulty or stressed needles can occasionally break; this is a very rare problem and to my knowledge has never resulted in the necessity for a surgical procedure to remove an imbedded piece of metal. On the one or two occasions that I have heard of needles breaking, they are usually simply removed with a pair of forceps.

The use of an electro-acupuncture stimulator is contraindicated if the patient has a cardiac pacemaker. As with transcutaneous nerve stimulation, electro-acupuncture stimulators may either switch off cardiac pacemakers or drive them at a dangerous rate. Other than this, the dangers of electro-acupuncture are the same as those of ordinary needling.

In conclusion, it would appear that acupuncture is a very safe procedure, providing the needles are properly cleaned and sterilised in the same way as any other piece of reusable surgical equipment, and the practitioner has a good basic knowledge of anatomy so he can avoid inserting needles into the lung or peritoneal cavity. Adverse reactions to pharmacological medications tend to be idiosyncratic. Damage caused by acupuncture is usually the product of inadequate training, thoughtlessness or incompetence on the part of the acupuncturist.

Transcutaneous electrical nerve stimulation (TENS)

Treatment with electrical stimulation for pain is not a new idea. The Romans used electric eels to provide shock therapy for arthritic patients, and the Victorians produced a large number of manually operated galvanic stimulation machines to treat a wide range of conditions. TENS involves the application of pulsed square-wave electrical current through surface electrodes placed on the skin. In all the epidemiological work published from general practice, pain is recorded as one of the most common presenting symptoms. Furthermore, analgesics are among the most commonly prescribed (or self-prescribed) medications. Pain is therefore a major problem for the general population, and TENS represents a valuable addition to the armamentarium of pain management. The major impetus and development of this technique came from a growing knowledge, during the late 1960s, of pain and its possible mechanisms. Melzack and Wall's gate control theory of pain suggested that it was at least theoretically possible that stimulation techniques could provide some degree of pain relief, and TENS, along with dorsal column stimulation, was one of the approaches suggested during the early 1970s. The putative mechanisms for TENS as an analgesic have already been discussed.

Clinical effectiveness

A number of controlled studies have been published which show that TENS is effective in the treatment of chronic pain. Melzack noted in 1975 that prolonged pain relief could be obtained by brief periods of stimulation with TENS; he studied 100 patients with chronic pain. More recently, a number of trials have been published which have evaluated the use of a functioning stimulator as compared with a defunctioned one.

- In these studies the defunctioned machines have been tampered with so that they look as if they work but in fact do not deliver a current to the patient (mock TENS); as already mentioned, these produce a placebo response of approximately 30%. The chronic pain states evaluated in this manner include low back pain, phantom limb pain, pain caused by osteoarthritis of the knee, and pain caused by rheumatoid arthritis. All these show that a functioning TENS machine is significantly more effective than a defunctioned one, and that the treatment is effective in approximately 45–50% of patients depending on the condition studied.

TENS has also been used to treat the pain caused by malignancy. The available descriptive studies suggest that it provides effective pain relief in about 50% of patients with malignant pain; extremity and trunk pain seem to respond more readily than perineal or pelvic pain. However, as the malignancy progresses, the analgesic effects may diminish and large doses of powerful drugs are usually required.

Analgesics will continue to provide the mainstay of therapy for acute transient pain states. However, TENS is of proven value in some types of acute pain, particularly postoperative and labour pain. A large study from Sweden has demonstrated that TENS is the only analgesic required by 70% of women in labour. From our knowledge of the natural history of labour pain, it is probable that even in a well-run and supportive obstetric unit, at least 80% of women will require some form of analgesia during labour and delivery. Studies on the obstetric use of TENS have also noted that neonatal Apgar scores are consistently higher in those mothers delivering with the aid of TENS alone. The reason being that the use of exogenous opiates such as pethidine almost invariably leads to respiratory depression in the neonate immediatly after delivery. Studies on postoperative pain relief have also demonstrated a clear decrease in the analgesic requirement during this period when TENS is used immediately postoperatively. Patients receiving TENS for postoperative pain seem to mobilise more swiftly and have fewer postoperative complications. Experimental support for the clinical effectiveness of TENS in acute pain has been provided by studies on experimentally induced dental pain, which show in an unambiguous manner that TENS can diminish the pain invoked by dental stimuli.

It is probable that TENS, like acupuncture, can be used to treat a wide range of non-painful conditions. The objective evidence for the efficacy of TENS in diseases such as asthma, anxiety and depression is minimal, and many further detailed studies will be required before we can make any real assessment of its efficacy in these conditions.

Adverse reactions

It is important to remember that before using any treatment for pain a clear diagnosis should be made, and the use of TENS is no exception to this rule. The treatment itself is surprisingly free from side-effects, although the machine should not be used if the patient has a cardiac pacemaker (it may switch it off) or while operating heavy machinery such as driving a car. The rubber electrodes are connected to the patient by the use of a electroconductive jelly. Allergic skin reactions to the electrode jelly have been reported, but these do not represent a major problem and are simply treated either by changing the jelly used or by the use of topical applications.

Acupuncture compared with TENS

Clinically TENS is probably less effective (by about 15–20%) than acupuncture. Studies that have compared these two therapies are few and far between and have often been designed with so few patients that it is not possible to reach firm conclusions. However, the overall picture from the clinical trials of acupuncture in pain gives the reader the impression of a 60% effective treatment rate; TENS studies report approximately a 45% effective treatment rate.

However, TENS is convenient, portable and often of value to patients in alleviating pain. In my experience, patients who respond to TENS almost invariably do well with acupuncture, but those who do well with acupuncture do not always respond to TENS.

If patients are given TENS for a limited period of time, then they usually find that symptoms return after a period of 1 or 2 months. This short-term pain relief can often be overcome by repeating treatment regularly. In comparable situations (such as the treatment of osteoarthritis of the knee) acupuncture appears to provide effective analgesia for a longer period, on average about 6 months. If the acupuncture is repeated, then a further prolonged period of pain relief is likely to occur. One of the main advantages of TENS is that the patients (if they have a machine) can treat themselves regularly, for as long as required. Acupuncture is usually a treatment that is effected by a therapist and consequently is provided less frequently and is more inconvenient from the patient's point of view. TENS is a fairly simple technique and the knowledge required for its effective use can be absorbed fairly swiftly by qualified medical or paramedical personnel. It requires a small amount of time to explain the technique to patients and a regular review of their progress. However the use of TENS is not as labour intensive as acupuncture for the therapist. It would appear that TENS could provide an effective, cheap, practical and relatively side-effect-free method of managing painful conditions.

Indications for the use of TENS

From the preceding discussion it is clear that TENS can be used, and is likely to be effective, in a wide range of painful conditions. There has been a tendency, particularly within the context of pain clinics, to use it as a 'last resort' treatment for intractable pain that has failed to respond to other therapies. Fortunately this attitude is changing and TENS is now used more as a first-line treatment in pain clinics, and is generally available in physiotherapy departments throughout the United Kingdom, but there are only few general practitioners in the United Kingdom who are using this therapy. In my opinion it would be extremely valuable to use TENS as an equivalent therapy to analgesics and non-steroidal anti-inflammatory agents for chronic pain, in the context of general practice, particularly in view of its minimal side-effects.

The following are some general guidelines that might be of help as indicators for the use of TENS.

1. Adverse reactions to analgesic or non-steroidal anti-inflammatory agents, for example gastrointestinal pathology or excessive drowsiness.

2. Failure to respond to drug therapy or potentially dangerous drug interactions if further analgesic therapy is required.

3. Patient preference: a patient may be in pain but for a variety of reasons may not wish to take prescribed drugs.

Parameters of stimulation

Probably the most difficult aspect of treatment with TENS is to know where to place the skin electrodes. The simplest and most practical guide is to place the electrodes on the point or points of greatest tenderness on, or around, the painful area. Some patients may experience a worsening of symptoms if the electrodes are placed on a neuralgic area. Occasionally a useful clinical effect can be obtained by placing the electrode pads just next to the spine, over the dermatome supplying the site of pain. The electrode pads may also be placed over acupuncture points, and the guidelines for the selection and use of body acupuncture points are directly applicable to electrode placement for TENS. Probably the most critical parameter in the use of TENS is the site of electrode placement, and sometimes small variations in this may produce a dramatic improvement in the clinical response.

Most machines available have one or two outputs supplying two or four electrode pads. It is often valuable to have a machine with four electrode pads as this allows a larger number of painful sites to be treated at any one session. All TENS machines have frequency and amplitude adjustments. The frequency in the majority of units varies from 2 to 200 hertz and the amplitude is often in the range of 0–50 mA into a 1-kΩ load. Unfortunately, ideal frequency adjustments to treat particular problems of specific patients have not been clearly defined, and obtaining the best frequency for an individual is often a matter of trial and error. In general it seems best to use high frequencies on local tender points, at least initially. The amplitude should be adjusted so that the patient feels a comfortable tingling sensation in the area of the skin electrodes; painful TENS does not seem to produce a better clinical result. Often one electrode is perceived as stronger, but this does not seem to have any proven clinical relevance. The TENS machine can be used two or three times a week for about an hour at each session, or almost continually. In general chronic pain will require more stimulation to obtain analgesia than minimal or acute pain.

Clinical response

The optimum values for stimulation and duration of therapy, for a particular patient, can only be realistically ascertained by lending the patient a machine for at least 2 or 3 weeks. I usually begin by explaining the machine to the patient in detail (which requires about 10 minutes consultation time) and connecting him or her to a machine to see whether it is functioning; I then leave the TENS on for about 30 minutes, disconnect it and send the patient home with it. The patient should then go away and try the machine out, in order to see whether a useful clinical effect can be obtained.

I usually advise patients to start off by using the machine for about half an hour twice a day and then alter the time of stimulation depending on the response obtained. The doctor should review the patient weekly to make sure that the machine is being used correctly, for instance to check that the batteries are still functioning. If no therapeutic benefit is gained in the first few sessions, then the patient should be encouraged to try placing the electrodes on different points and also try using different frequencies.

The patient's pain may respond in one of three ways: no improvement, dramatic improvement, and slow but sure improvement. If after trying the machine for 2 or 3 weeks no improvement has been obtained, it is unlikely that this technique will provide effective analgesia. If the patient is obtaining slow improvement, then the analgesic effect will usually increase progressively in direct proportion to the length of time of treatment. A swift, dramatic improvement occurs occasionally, and this usually means that treatment needs to be repeated infrequently in order to obtain an effective clinical response. Very occasionally a slight worsening of symptoms may occur and this usually means either that there will be no response or that the patient has had too much treatment. The patient should therefore be advised to stop using the machine for a few days and see if the condition improves. If the patient does improve, then the machine should be used occasionally.

Obtaining TENS machines

This process will vary from country to country depending on the local system of health care provision. In the United Kingdom only a few patients can obtain TENS machines for their own personal use through the National Health Service, usually through pain clinics where regional finance is set aside for the purchase of a large number of machines that are on permanent or semi-permanent loan. If general practitioners wish to purchase a TENS machine, they have to buy it through their own general practice fund; this therapy is not available on prescription. A good guide to the equipment available in the United Kingdom can be obtained from the Department of Medical Physics, Hallamshire Hospital, Sheffield. Anyone thinking of using TENS will need to purchase a machine so that it can be lent to patients. If the machines prove clinically effective, then the therapist can request a patient to buy his own machine in order to obtain more permanent benefit from the therapy.

Conclusion

TENS is a simple and effective analgesic therapy. Although the evidence strongly suggests that it is significantly less effective than acupuncture, it does have many advantages. It can be used by patients to manage their own problems, and therefore a little investment in time and explanation as to how to use the machine may pay dividends in the management of a chronic problem. Furthermore, the patient will not suffer the side-effects frequently induced by other analgesic therapies.

Obtaining acupuncture treatment

There are three groups of acupuncturists in the United Kingdom: lay acupuncturists, medically qualified acupuncturists, and physiotherapists. There are many excellent non-medically qualified acupuncturists, although inevitably there are some of a poor standard. It is now possible for a registered medical practitioner to refer a patient to a non-medically qualified person; however, the medical practitioner must retain responsibility for the continuing care of that patient. Therefore, before recommending or referring the patient to a lay acupuncturist, it is essential that a clear diagnosis should be made by the referring doctor, who should have some detailed knowledge of the qualifications and standard of practice of the lay acupuncturist to whom he is referring the patient.

The names and addresses of the majority of medically qualified acupuncturists can be obtained through the British Medical Acupuncture Society. This is an organisation of registered medical and dental practitioners, and full members are all practising acupuncturists. Any medical person can refer a patient directly to a member of the British Medical Acupuncture Society in the same way that he would refer a patient to another doctor for any treatment.

Recently physiotherapists have begun to train in acupuncture for the relief of pain. At present there are only a small number practising acupuncture, but this is likely to grow in the future. The guidelines for physiotherapists practising acupuncture are the same as those for physiotherapists practising manipulation, or indeed any other form of physical therapy. The treatment provided by physiotherapists is usually either requested by a doctor or suggested by the physiotherapist in consultation with the referring doctor. It is probable that through the assistance of a growing band of properly trained physiotherapists, acupuncture may become widely available within the National Health Service.

Acupuncture courses

A list of recognised teachers is provided by the British Medical Acupuncture Society (see below). A number of courses are run in the United Kingdom, which teach a wide range of different approaches to acupuncture. Anyone thinking of going on an acupuncture course should, in my opinion, make sure that the course they wish to attend has some practical input. Ideally this should involve the course participants needling patients under the clinical supervision of an experienced practitioner. The courses offered by Members of the British Medical Acupuncture Society are in general exclusively for medically qualified personnel.

The Chartered Society of Physiotherapy (see below) can be contacted about courses approved as a part of the physiotherapists' continuing postgraduate education.

A number of courses are available to non-medical or para-medically qualified people; information about these can be obtained from the British Acupuncture Association and the College of Traditional Chinese Acupuncture (see below).

References

Akil H., Richardson D., Hughes J., Barchas J. (1976). Antagonism of stimulation-produced analgesia by naloxone, A. Narcotic antagonist. *Science*; **191**:961–2.

Becker R. (1974). The significances of bio-electric potentials. *Bioelectrochemistry and Bioenergetics*; **1**:187–99.

Becker R., Reichmanis M., Marino A., Spadaro J. (1976). Electrophysiological correlates of acupuncture points and meridians. *Psycho-energetic Systems*; **1**:105–12.

Chang H. T. (1973). Integrative action of the thalamus in the process of acupuncture for analgesia. *Scientia Sinia*; **16**:25–60.

Chapman C., Benedetti C., Colpitts Y., Gerlach R. (1983). Naloxone fails to reserve pain thresholds elevated by acupuncture; acupuncture analgesia reconsidered. *Pain*; **16**:13–31.

Chapman C., Sato T., Martin R., Tanaka A., Okazaki N., Colpitts Y., Mayeno J., Gagliardi G. (1982). Comparative effects of acupuncture in Japan and the United States on dental pain perception. *Pain*; **12**:319–28.

Chen-Yu, Jen-Yi, Teh-Hsing, Yao-Hui, Shu-Chieh (1975). Studies of spinal ascending pathways for the effect of acupuncture analgesia in rabbits. *Scientia Sinia*; **17**:651–8.

Clement-Jones V., McLoughlin L., Lowry P., Besser G., Rees L., Wen L. (1979). Acupuncture and heroin addicts; changes in met-enkephalin and beta-endorphin in blood and cerebrospinal fluid. *Lancet*; **2**:380–82.

Dupont A., Barden N., Cusan L., Merand Y., Labrie F., Vaudry H.

(1980). Beta-endorphin and met-enkephalins; their distribution, modulation by oestrogens and haloperidol and role in a neuro-endocrine control. *Federation Proceedings*; **39**:2544–50.

Hughes J., Smith T., Kosterlitz H., Fothergill L., Morgan B., Morriss H. (1975). Identification of two related pentapeptides from the brain with potent opiate agonist activity. *Nature*; **258**:577–9.

Jisheng H. (1979). The role of some central neurotransmitters in acupuncture analgesia. *National Symposium of Acupuncture Moxibustion and Acupuncture Anaesthesia*, pp. 27–30. Peking: Foreign Language Press.

Ke-Fi, Shu-Fang (1977). Effect of stimulation of bulbar reticular formation on long latency discharges in the region of the nucleus centralis lateralis of the thalamus. *Scientia Sinia*; **20**:475–81.

Kenyon J. N. (1983). *Modern Techniques of Acupuncture*, Vol. II, pp. 13–42. Wellingborough: Thorsons.

Le Bars D., Dickenson A., Besson J. M. (1979). Diffuse noxious inhibitory controls. Part I. Effects on dorsal horn convergent neurones in the rat. Part II. Lack of effect on non-convergent neurones, supra-spinal involvement and theoretical implications. *Pain*; **6**:283–327.

Lewith G., Machin D. (1983). On the evaluation of the clinical effects of acupuncture. *Pain*; **16**:111–27.

Mann F. (1977). *Scientific Aspects of Acupuncture*, pp. 1–29. London: Heinemann Medical.

Melzack R. (1975). Prolonged relief of pain by brief intense transcutaneous somatic stimulation. *Pain*; **1**:357–74.

Melzack R., Stillwell P., Fox D. (1977). Trigger points and acupuncture points for pain; correlations and implications. *Pain*; **3**:3–23.

Melzack R., Wall P. (1965). Pain mechanisms, a new theory. *Science*; **150**:971–9.

Nathan P., Rudge P. (1974). Testing the gate control theory of pain in man. *Journal of Neurology, Neurosurgery and Psychiatry*; **37**:1366–72.

National Symposium of Acupuncture Moxibustion and Acupuncture Anaesthesia (1979). Peking: Foreign Language Press.

Oleson T. D., Kroening J. R., Bresler D. E. (1980). An experimental evaluation of auricular diagnosis; the somatotopic mapping of musculoskeletal pain at ear acupuncture points. *Pain*; **8**:217–29.

Pomeranz B. (1981). Acupuncture analgesia. In *Persistent Pain*, Vol. III (Lipton, S., ed.) pp. 241–58. London: Academic Press.

Pomeranz B., Chiu D. (1976). Naloxone blocks acupuncture analgesia and causes hyperalgesia. *Life Sciences*, **19**:1757–62.

Sjolund B., Trenius L., Eriksson M. (1977). Increased cerebrospinal fluid levels of endorphins after electro-acupuncture. *Acta Physiologica Scandinavica*; **100**:382–4.

Suggested reading

Anon. (1980). *Essentials of Chinese Acupuncture*. Peking: Foreign Language Press.

Ersek R. A. (1981). *Pain Control with TENS, Principles and Practice*. St. Louis, Miss.: Warren H. Green.

Kenyon J. (1983). *Modern Techniques of Acupuncture*, Vols. I and II. Wellingborough: Thorsons. (Vol. III in press.)

Lewith G. T., Lewith N. R. (1980). *Electrode Placement for Transcutaneous Electrical Nerve Stimulation; a Method Based on Classical Body Acupuncture*. Croydon: R.D.G. Electro-Medical.

Lewith G. T., Lewith N. R. (1983). *Modern Chinese Acupuncture*, 2nd edn. Wellingborough: Thorsons.

Lu Gwei-Djen, Needham J. (1980). *Celestial Lancets*. Cambridge: Cambridge University Press.

Porkert M. (1978). *The Theoretical Foundations of Chinese Medicine*. London: MIT Press.

Veith I., ed. (1972). *The Yellow Emperor's Classic of Internal Medicine (Nei Ching Su Wen)*. University of California Press.

Note. Essentials of Chinese Acupuncture and *The Yellow Emperor's Classic of Internal Medicine* do not have defined authors.

Useful addresses

British Medical Acupuncture Society
67–69 Chancery Lane
London WC2 1AF.

Chartered Society of Physiotherapy
14 Bedford Row
London WC1R 4ED.

British Acupuncture Association
34 Alderney Street
London SW1B 4EU.

The College of Traditional Chinese Acupuncture
Tao House
Queensway
Royal Leamington Spa
Warwickshire CV31 3LZ.

The Centre for the Study of Alternative Therapies
51 Bedford Place
Southampton SO1 2DG.

Chapter 2

Manipulation
P. Wells

Definition

The word 'manipulation' is derived from the Latin verb *manipulare*, to handle, its general sense being conveyed by the use of the hands in a skilful manner. In the context of therapy it has been defined specifically as skilful or dextrous treatment by the hand.

Many procedures are grouped under the generic title 'manipulation', but each of them involves some form of movement of the patient's tissues by the operator. This is done while the patient remains relaxed and in a purely passive role. By contrast, 'exercise' is active and involves effort and voluntary movement by the patient.

Relaxation by the person receiving manipulative treatment is essential, first, in order that the manipulator may accurately judge the mobility of the joints, muscles and ligaments, and second, that their response to what is being done may be assessed with precision before, during and after any procedure.

Manipulative techniques are applied in treating the musculoskeletal system when pain and restricted movement, or occasionally excessive movement, have resulted from trauma, degenerative change and postural stress. Both spinal as well as peripheral joints and their associated tissues are treatable by these procedures.

Classification of manipulative techniques

The subject of manipulation is bedevilled by semantics. The word itself, to those who practise the art, covers a wide range of procedures from the very gentle to the more firm or vigorous. Amongst those knowing little or nothing of the subject, and that includes most of the general public, the impression sometimes exists that it involves overforceful and aggressive manoeuvres. Many who are medically qualified associate manipulation with high-velocity thrust techniques and little else. One grouping of manipulative procedures includes all the techniques of massage. It is clear that 'manipulation' may mean different things to different people, but it is commonly taken to mean a procedure carried out at high speed as a short-amplitude thrust applied to a joint or series of joints. The expression 'manipulative procedures', on the other hand, encompasses a much wider range of passive movement techniques. Clearly we require some framework in which we can categorise the many procedures which are commonly employed. Such a framework, now used, for example, by most physiotherapists, is as follows.

1. Soft tissue techniques.
2. Regional mobilisation.
3. Localised mobilisation.
4. Regional manipulation.
5. Localised manipulation.

We should be clear what we mean by each of these categories.

To start with, what is the difference between 'mobilisation' and 'manipulation'? 'Mobilisation' consists of passive movement techniques usually employing repetitive movement, which is under the patient's control. By this we mean that if the patient for any reason communicates to the operator that he wishes the technique to be stopped, then it can be. The patient is, of course, relaxed throughout and does not control what happens by any active movement on his part. Repetitive oscillatory movements to relax muscles, relieve pain or carefully elongate tight structures come under the grouping of 'mobilisation'.

A 'manipulation', on the other hand, consists of a single, high-velocity thrust applied to a joint or series of joints and soft tissues. This procedure gaps or moves the joint very quickly and is carried out to create extra freedom of movement and to relieve pain. Because of its speed and the fact that it is only ever attempted while the patient is relaxed, the technique is not under the patient's control. It is over almost before he knows it has been done.

We may now therefore define broadly the categories we have set down.

Soft tissue techniques (Fig. 2.1)

These consist of a range of procedures, sometimes grouped together as 'massage'. There is a tendency now to use the expression 'soft tissue techniques' since the word 'massage' has come to acquire a very general and non-medical connotation. This is a pity since good massage administered by a skilled and medically trained expert can give very beneficial results in a number of conditions, especially orthopaedic and rheumatological ones.

Although massage of various sorts has always been on offer from an assortment of non-medical masseuses, ranging from the poorly trained to the very adept, recently the number seems to have mushroomed. This growth in the popularity of generalised and non-specific massage aimed at helping the individual to relax has seen a decline in the use of massage by those who are properly medically trained such as physiotherapists. The other more important reason why the use of massage on a large scale by those medically trained has declined is that recent decades have seen the growth of our knowledge of joint and soft tissue neurology and biomechanics. As a result it is becoming clear that many problems previously thought to arise principally within the soft tissues such as muscles do in fact owe more of their cause to joint disturbances. They then manifest themselves secondarily in muscles, fascia and so forth. 'Fibrositis' is a good example. This may seem like splitting hairs, but it is an important factor in explaining why more attention is placed now than hitherto on analysing very specifically the joint and movement abnormalities underlying the problem and why less emphasis is given to treating purely the soft tissue disturbances accompanying it. Nonetheless, soft tissue or massage techniques maintain their rightful place in the field of natural medical alternatives to drug therapy and surgery and are taught to physiotherapists at both pre- and postgraduate levels. It is just that their use is now restricted to very specific instances when they are judged to be particularly beneficial.

Regional mobilisation (Fig. 2.2)

Whereas trauma and degenerative change frequently give rise to very localised and specific musculoskeletal problems, generalised 'stiffness' and regional disturbances in movement do also arise. This may sometimes occur in the spine, for example,

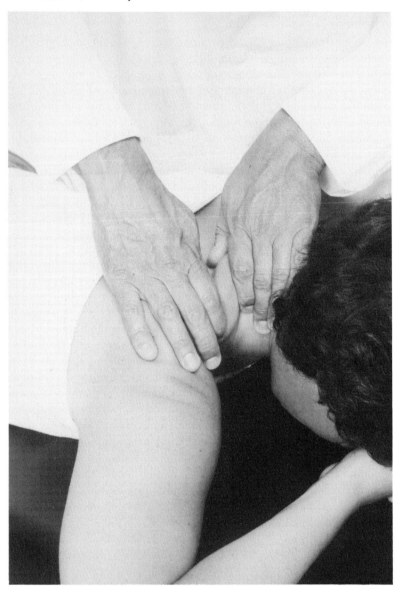

Fig. 2.1 *Soft tissue technique to stretch and relax the upper fibres of the trapezius and levator scapulae muscles. Such techniques are useful to mobilise the tight, sore tissues which are often found with chronic joint problems.*

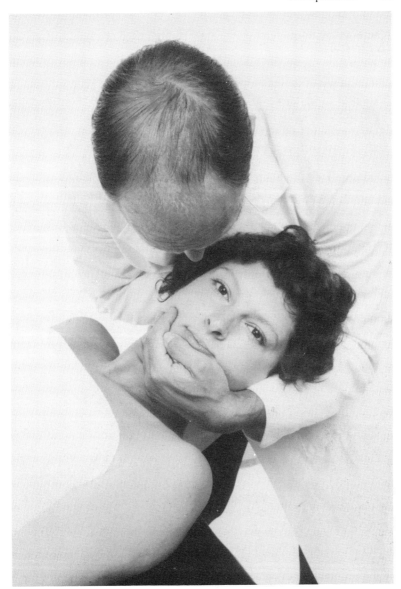

Fig. 2.2 A rotational mobilisation procedure for the cervical spine. By positioning the appropriate level of the neck midway between flexion and extension the generalised technique can emphasise motion at that level. The movement is a repetitive oscillatory one, carried out through a prescribed arc of the available range of cervical rotation, invariably away from the painful side.

where many small movements are summated from a large number of joints to give each particular spinal region its characteristic freedom of movement.

It is in such situations that regional mobilisation techniques are used which affect a group of joints and their soft tissues. At the same time, by careful positioning, it is possible to direct the effects of regional mobilisation to a particular spinal level if this is considered necessary.

Included in this category is traction, a stretching force which is applied in general along the longitudinal axis of the tissues. The precise magnitude of the traction force, the position in which it is given, and the time for which it is carried out may all bear upon its effect and so it is important to administer traction in a very accurate and predetermined way. This is best carried out with specialised apparatus devised to do just that (Figs. 2.3 and 2.4). However, such 'mechanical' traction is still clearly within the field of manipulation since the tissues of the body are passively moved, albeit in this case by a traction machine rather than by operator's hands.

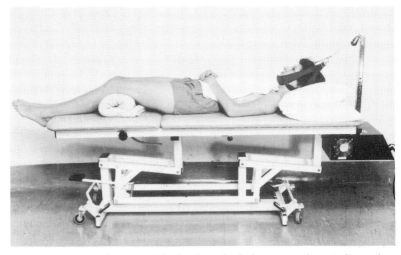

Fig 2.3 Cervical traction. The level to which the tractive force is directed is determined by the degree of flexion of the head-upon-neck or neck-upon-trunk. In this instance, the cervico-thoracic junction is being treated. Motorised traction may be used to apply a sustained (not the same as constant) or intermittent force to take into account the varying degrees of pain or stiffness to be treated. The upper thoracic levels can be treated with a similar arrangement.

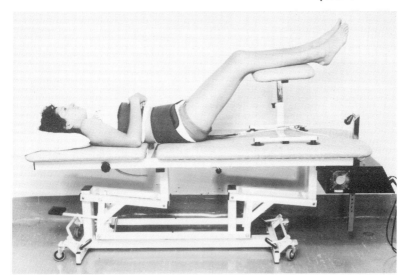

Fig. 2.4 Lumbar traction. The degree of hip flexion is used to determine the mid position of the relevent lumbar vertebral level being treated, and the legs are supported accordingly. Sustained or intermittent traction can be given as with the cervical spine. The lower thoracic levels can be treated with some modifications in positioning of the patient and the harnesses.

Localised mobilisation (Fig. 2.5)

Just as it is common to find some specific problem localised to one or another peripheral joint such as the shoulder or knee, so it is very common to be able to locate a vertebral problem to a specific level of the spine. In those situations localised mobilisation (as distinct from manipulation) is employed to move the mobility segment at fault in a carefully controlled way. A mobility segment can be defined as the moveable junction between two adjacent vertebral segments (e.g. L5 and S1), including their associated joints and soft tissues.

While every attempt is made to localise forces with great care to the level being treated, no manipulative procedure can ever be entirely localised since the adjacent levels are bound to move somewhat also. Even so, it comes as a surprise to many observers to see how accurate such techniques can be in the hands of a skilled and experienced manipulative therapist.

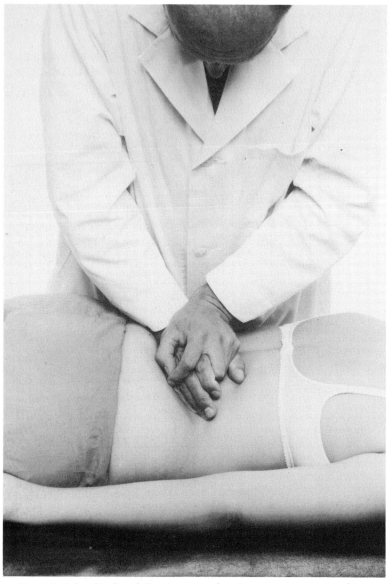

Fig. 2.5 *A localised mobilisation procedure in a postero-anterior direction being performed at the fourth lumbar vertebral level. A small but definite range of accessory movement can be obtained, localised by a small area of the hypothenar eminence of the underneath hand. The movement may be a sustained or an oscillatory one.*

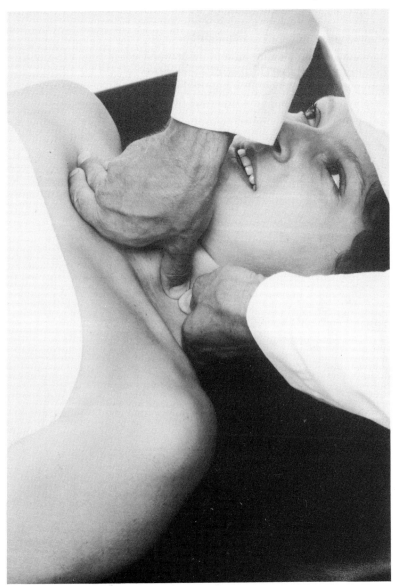

Fig. 2.6 *A localised cervical mobilisation procecure being performed unilaterally in an antero-posterior direction. Contact is being maintained with the front of the transverse process of the vertebra. A carefully graded accessory movement is performed either gently or more firmly into the range of movement, as appropriate.*

Regional manipulation (Fig. 2.6)

The majority of joint problems resolve with the use of regional or localised mobilisations and do not need a manipulative thrust technique. In the case of spinal dysfunction, about 15–20% of patients generally require one or more 'manipulations' to clear their symptoms and restore good functional movement.

If the restriction of movement affects a number of adjacent mobility segments in the spine, then a regional manipulation may be used. By careful positioning and control fundamental to all manipulative procedures these high-velocity techniques of controlled amplitude can effectively regain movement simultaneously at a number of adjacent levels.

Localised manipulation (Figs. 2.7 and 2.8)

When mobilisation has failed to gain completely the degree of joint mobility reasonably expected, it may be necessary to carry

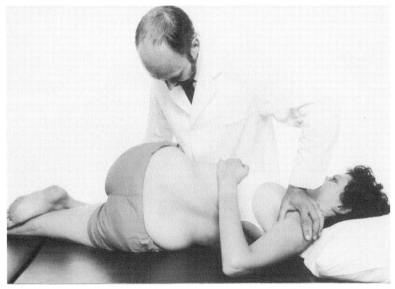

Fig. 2.7 A generalised rotational manipulation for the mid to lower lumbar spine. Such a procedure is usually performed to improve the local signs and symptoms arising form regional stiffness in the low back. Even though a the force and amplitude are carefully controlled, such a procedure would not be used in the presence of a segmentel hypermobility within the area.

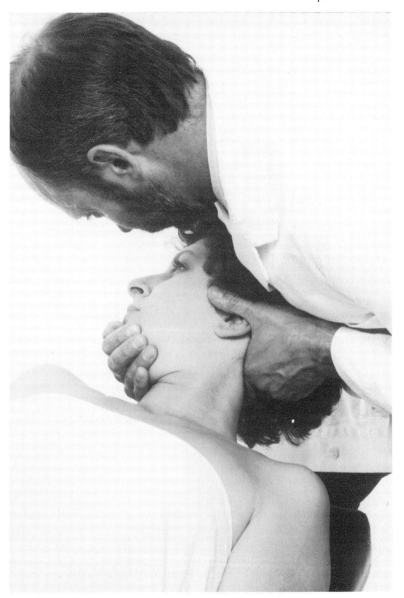

Fig. 2.8 *A localised postero-anterior thrust technique to mobilise the left atlanto-occipital joint. The cervical spine is well short of full rotation and a small direct thrust with the left hand directed through the plane of the joint achieves the movement.*

out a localised manipulation. By careful positioning and a very precise application of the force used, either with short or long leverage, a degree of movement can be obtained suddenly at a joint previously abnormally tight and restricted. The speed employed is crucial in most cases, both in the application of the force and in its release, for a successful manipulation. The amplitude of the movement used is always small and very controlled, as part of the built-in safety of each manoeuvre. Great skill is required to carry out localised manipulation successfully and such skill takes much time and practice to acquire.

It is doubtful whether any localised manipulation is ever as entirely localised as the title suggests. Even with the most skilful and careful positioning and force application, adjacent joints and tissues invariably receive some of the stress imparted by the technique. The point is that this is minimal when expertly carried out and of course far more localised than a generalised manipulation seeks to be.

Manipulation under anaesthetic (MUA)

There may come a point in treatment when mobilisation and manipulation cease to improve the situation further or when progress is exceedingly slow. At this stage the surgeon or physician in overall charge of the patient may decide that a manipulation of the spinal level or peripheral joint concerned should be carried out under an anaesthetic. Whereas that decision is the doctor's alone, it will usually be made after consultation with the physiotherapist who has been carrying out the treatment. Dr James Cyriax (1978) has recorded the indications for the technique. Obviously that which can be achieved while the patient is conscious and able to respond is preferable to a procedure performed while the individual is anaesthetised and cannot react. The subjective and objective responses to any manoeuvre are what guides treatment and the degree of gentleness or vigour used. Conscious subjects can report changes in their symptoms immediately, and objective testing likewise will give essential information quickly. However, if fibrosis in the soft tissues of the joint is so dense that a firm manoeuvre is required which would be too uncomfortable for the unanaesthetised patient, or if the patient is unable to relax or is of a body build which prevents the procedure from being carried out, then the use of an anaesthetic may provide a way forward.

The use of this technique has been criticised on the grounds that it is like taking a sledgehammer to crack a nut. However, when used sparingly and for specific indications the results may be seen to justify the means. Cyriax (1978) considers the procedure to be contraindicated in the cervical and thoracic regions.

Maitland (1977) has pointed out that 'follow-up' physiotherapy is only indicated if the symptoms have not responded sufficiently to the MUA. If complete relief of symptoms is gained, then follow-up treatment is unnecessary. He also makes the following important observation: 'Where manipulation of the conscious patient has failed, MUA may be successful. The converse is also true. Sometimes ... patients may require a balance of both.'

Alternative medicine

The only sense in which manipulation should now be considered 'alternative' is when it is used instead of drugs and surgery. Frequently, manipulative treatment is used as an adjunct to drugs or surgery. Commonly, at least where manipulative doctors and physiotherapists are concerned, manipulation is employed on an empirical basis within the context of orthodox medicine to treat a very wide range of musculoskeletal disorders. However, it is still common to hear the belief expressed that manipulation is an alternative to orthodox medical treatment and is only therefore ever available 'outside' and from those non-medically qualified. This lingering belief is historical and from that point of view is understandable. It is changing, however, to the more accurate observation that manipulation is now far more widely available than ever before within 'orthodox' medicine as well as outside it.

Large numbers of doctors and physiotherapists, specially trained and highly skilled, employ manipulative procedures as an intrinsic part of their day-to-day management of spinal and peripheral joint and soft tissue problems. They include those who work in National Health Service hospitals, sports clinics, general practice, private practice and industrial medicine.

The large body of manual therapists and the increasing number of medical and surgical colleagues who refer patients to them for their specialist skills, are steadily making the public more aware that this logical and effective treatment is available where it belongs, within the field of orthodox medicine. The art and science of manipulation have been transferred back into the mainstream of Western medicine where it had its early beginnings.

Historical background

An excellent history of manipulation is available in Schiotz and Cyriax (1975) and therefore only a brief outline is given here.

Early history

The use of manipulation, particularly in treating spinal disorders, has a long history. It was recorded in a description on the treatment of lumbar kyphosis by Hippocrates, the Greek father of medicine, as far back as 400 BC. In a chapter entitled *Peri arthron* (*About joints*) a method of reducing a lumbar kyphosis is described in which the patient, lying prone, is stretched by assistants at the head and feet while the physician presses on the prominent vertebrae with the hands, foot or body weight. The use of a padded board levered across the back is given as an alternative method, considered the more effective by Hippocrates.

The great physician Galen (AD 131–202) quotes Hippocrates' methods and also describes a case of a man who, following an accident, developed paraesthesiae and numbness in the third, fourth and fifth fingers of the hand. He ascribed the injury to the 'spinal nerve below the seventh cervical vertebra' and recounts how the patient was cured by treatment of his neck.

Avicenna, the Arabian physician (AD 980–1037) who practised at a hospital in Baghdad, used the manipulative methods of Hippocrates in the treatment of back problems. Illustrations in a later sixteenth century Latin transcription of his great work the *Canon Avicennae* show the method of using sustained pressure or thrust during spinal traction to treat 'a dislocation outwards of the lumbar vertebra'. The same methods continued to be advocated throughout the Renaissance period in Europe and into the seventeenth century.

Bone setters

Accounts exist from many countries and cultures, including

Europe and America, of individuals employing rudimentary manipulation to treat those suffering from limb or spinal injuries. As far back as the seventeenth century, for example, a bone setter was employed at St Bartholomew's Hospital in London (Schiotz and Cyriax, 1975).

These 'bone setters' were so named because of their claim that their skills repositioned bones which had become displaced. Almost every village and most towns, it would seem, had such a healer. Usually the skill ran through a family and was handed on from one generation to the next; the family might be that of a local farmer or blacksmith. Considerable controversy surrounded the bone setters and permeated the medical establishment in the second-half of the nineteenth century and on into the early decades of this. These lay manipulators, practising without any formal medical education, drew constant criticism from the surgeons and physicians of the day, many of whom no doubt saw the disastrous results of some of their handiwork.

While the wise recognised the undoubted benefit from their successful and no doubt sometimes very skilful treatment, the practice of manipulation gained a bad name by and large. Fuel was added to the fire by the formation just before the turn of the century of the system of diagnosis and treatment called osteopathy, and a little later chiropractic. The founders of these schools in America and their followers set their faces squarely against the established medical system of diagnosis and treatment. Their claims to cure such conditions as diabetes, gall-stones, appendicitis and goitres by a number of treatments including various sorts of spinal manipulation placed them beyond the pale. In retrospect many of the criticisms of the doctors were well founded. Such conditions cannot be cured by spinal manipulation. Yet a great array of mechanical joint and soft tissue problems were treated successfully by these unorthodox practitioners. Their success endeared them to some doctors who acknowledged with magnanimity that they offered a large number of sufferers an effective treatment not taught or recognised within medicine at that time. The majority of doctors, however, in rejecting the more bizarre claims of these rival healers, also rejected and outlawed much of the good that the skilful and discerning ones did in practice. Manipulation as a concept and practice was equated with charlatanism by the majority of the medical profession.

Even so, a surgeon as eminent as Sir Robert Jones could make the following observation in 1931 (Gray, 1938).

...manipulation is a branch of surgery that from time immemorial has been neglected by our profession, and, as a direct consequence, much of it has fallen into the hands of the unqualified practitioner. Let there be no mistake; this has seriously undermined the public confidence, which has on occasions amounted to open hostility. If we honestly face the facts, this attitude should cause us no surprise. No excuse will avail us when a stiff joint, which has been treated for many months by various surgeons and practitioners without effect, rapidly regains its mobility and function at the hands of an irregular practitioner. We should be self-critical, and ask why we missed such an opportunity ourselves. The problem is not solved by pointing out mistakes made by the unqualified—the question at issue is their success. Reputations are not made in any walk of life simply by failures. Failures are common to us all, and it is a far wiser and more dignified attitude on our part to improve our armamentarium than dwell upon the mistakes made by others.

More recently, a few of the battle lines have melted away. Some of the claims of those within the manipulative groups once considered highly unorthodox have become more modest. At the same time developments within the fields of neurology, biomechanics and psychology have lent support to reasonable hypotheses which may be tested in support of manipulative treatment. So a more rational approach is now possible.

Who manipulates?

Manipulation is not confined to one profession or group of individuals, it is practised by doctors, physiotherapists, osteopaths, chiropractors and others. In order that it should be both safe and effective, it is essential that those who use it have sufficient general medical background to understand fully how pain and disease manifest themselves. There are both indications and contraindications for this form of treatment, and the manipulator must be thoroughly conversant with them.

The fundamental requirements common to all good manipulative practitioners are:

(a) that they carefully and thoroughly examine and assess the patient; and

(b) that they then use passive movement in one way or another to improve the patient's symptoms and signs.

Having highlighted those broad similarities, any attempt to go further and define the differences that separate the various manipulative groups becomes a daunting task. The general public and much of the medical world share in the general confusion about what distinguishes the theory and practice of the manipulation as used by manipulative physiotherapists, doctors, osteopaths and chiropractors. The task of explaining the differences is not made easier by the fact that within these professions one may discover a range of belief and practice related to manipulation.

The medical manipulator

This term may be used to distinguish the orthodox practitioner of medicine who, being a qualified doctor, then undergoes training and thereafter uses manipulation in his treatment of his patients. Whether the practitioner is an orthopaedic surgeon, a rheumatologist or a general practitioner, he may decide to use this approach to the patient's problem on its own or in combination with drugs such as analgesics, anti-inflammatories, antidepressants and so forth. Other measures such as epidural injection and manipulation under anaesthetic may also be used on occasions.

A doctor may choose to follow the system and methods of one particular group such as, for example, that of orthopaedic medicine whose principal protagonist is Dr James Cyriax. Alternatively, he may undertake training based upon a number of differing 'schools', selecting and using what he finds to be the most appropriate in his circumstances.

Medical manipulators, many of whom are in general practice, wish to use manipulative techniques in their day-to-day practice chiefly to treat patients suffering from a variety of benign, mechanical spinal disorders.

Manipulation by physiotherapists

Physiotherapy is the treatment of disease and disability by physical methods, and physiotherapists have always provided an alternative treatment to the drugs and surgery employed by the doctors alongside whom they practise. The use of passive movement procedures as well as active exercise has been built into the profession as an integral aspect of its work since its inception. Physiotherapists acquire refined manual skills from the earliest time in their training, and massage, mobilisation and manipulation are incorporated into the treatment of a wide variety of spinal and peripheral joint and soft tissue problems.

Many go on to specialise in the treatment of musculoskeletal problems and undertake more advanced courses in the management of these problems, including the use of manipulative techniques. All physiotherapists, even those in private practice, in industry, in sports medicine and so forth, work in close liaison with the patient's referring doctor and through those medical colleagues have access to detailed information about the patient's medical history. However, physiotherapists are trained never to undertake treatment of any sort unless they have carried out a thorough and comprehensive examination and assessment of the patient.

Whatever the emphasis given in any particular case to the use of manipulative procedures, these are always considered alongside such things as the need for muscle re-education, relaxation, postural re-alignment and careful education of the patient. There is evidence that a combination of such treatments is more effective than the use of any one of them alone (Coxhead *et al.*, 1981).

Like doctors, physiotherapists may adhere to the concepts and approach of one particular teacher and practitioner, such as Geoffrey Maitland, or they may undertake post-registration courses in a number of approaches, incorporating them into their practice as seems suitable. Today it is the general practice, in contrast to former years, for physiotherapists to select the treatments they use for each particular patient, having first received a diagnosis and a request for treatment from the referring surgeon or physician.

Chiropractors

In an article concerned with the history of the development of chiropractic concepts, Janse (1975) quotes four contemporary definitions of chiropractic.

1. Chiropractic is the study of problems of health and disease from a structural point of view with special consideration given to spinal mechanics and neurological relations, presenting the hypotheses that:
   (a) disease may be caused or aggravated by disturbances of the nervous system,
   (b) disturbances of the nervous system may be caused by derangements of the musculoskeletal structures.
2. Chiropractic is a discipline of the scientific healing arts concerned with the pathogenesis, diagnostics, therapeutics and prophylaxis of functional disturbances, pathomechanical states, pain syndromes and neurophysiological effects related to the statics and dynamics of the locomotor system, especially of the spine and pelvis.
3. Chiropractic is the science concerned with defects in the mechanics, statics and dynamics of the human body.
4. A definition by exclusion relates to chiropractic as 'the system or method of treating human ailments without the use of drugs or medicines and without operative surgery'.

One of the pivotal points in chiropraxy is the concept of spinal subluxation, which chiropractors define as a disrelationship or misalignment of adjacent spinal articulations. As a result of such subluxations, and the vascular and neurological changes which they postulate follow from them, chiropractors believe that not only musculoskeletal dysfunction will arise but also that disease in the various organ systems of the body may ensue. Thus chiropractic spinal 'adjustments' and manipulation become a treatment for diseases other than those of strictly mechanical musculoskeletal origin.

To quote Janse: 'It is for this reason that it is important and necessary that in the overall management of patients with visceral symptoms and if only to break up aberrant cycles, manipulative therapy be made available, if necessary, in collaboration with physicians of other disciplines.'

Examination includes the use of radiographs which are subject to complex analysis to identify 'intersegmental disrelationships'. Treatment, which usually includes specific 'adjustment', aims to restore normal alignment of the vertebral structures and pelvis.

The chiropractic adjustment is a specific form of direct articular manipulation utilising a short lever and characterised by a dynamic, forceful, high-velocity thrust of controlled amplitude.

Chiropractors in Britain work entirely in the private field, taking and interpreting their own radiographs and making their own diagnoses.

Osteopaths

Osteopathy is a system of diagnosis and treatment which pays special regard to the treatment of pain and dysfunction arising within the musculoskeletal system. At the same time it places great emphasis on the relationship between musculoskeletal lesions or somatic dysfunction and disturbances or disease of the viscera. Osteopaths believe that a somatic dysfunction, particularly when it affects structures such as the spinal apophyseal joints, is capable of producing changes in other body systems.

Northrup (1975) has stated:

Essentially, a somatic dysfunction (osteopathic lesion) of the synovial joint is a biomechanical process occurring in the musculoskeletal system with structural–functional changes occurring in the articular and peri-articular tissues resulting in subjective and/or objective signs and symptoms.

The manifestations of these biomechanical lesions are mediated through the neuro-circulatory system and may appear local to the lesion, in segmentally related but remote portions of the musculoskeletal system or as functional disturbances in other body systems.

Joint dysfunction can occur either from other somatic lesions or from visceral dysfunction or both.

Osteopaths use manipulation both to maintain normal function and to correct dysfunction, but emphasise that it is incorporated within the totality of the philosophy of osteopathy and not as a thing set apart.

While the concepts of osteopathy seem very similar to those of chiropractic, there are differences. Also, the techniques employed by the two groups differ, particularly the specific methods used to carry out manipulative thrust techniques. Like chiropractors, osteopaths in Britain work entirely within the private sphere.

Although manipulation forms the major treatment method of both osteopaths and chiropractors, these professions also make use of other approaches such as muscle re-education and the correction of postural faults. During their training they acquire great skills in manipulative technique. However, whereas some doctors do refer some of their patients to these practitioners and a few even go on themselves to train in their methods and ideas, a great divide still separates them from the majority in the medical world. Some of this separation may be due to the fact that old ideas and prejudices are very slow to die, but there still remain within chiropraxy and osteopathy concepts which those outside of their discipline find difficult to accept. For example, the chiropractors claim that most spinal problems are related to one or other vertebra being out of place or subluxated, and that these can be repositioned is unacceptable to most doctors and non-chiropractic manipulators.

It is often when such concepts and the dogmatic attitudes which uphold them are scrutinised that the antagonism between manipulative 'schools' becomes evident. Until such ideas see the full light of day and are openly put forward and discussed to separate what is reasonable from what seems patent nonsense, a big divide will continue to exist between 'orthodox' manipulators and the 'non-orthodox' ones.

What is treatable by manipulation?

A large and varied range of ailments whose origins lie in some dysfunction or malfunctioning of musculoskeletal structures are amenable to carefully selected and suitably modified manipulative treatment. Under the heading 'musculoskeletal structures' come the joints and all their associated soft tissues such as ligaments and joint capsules, muscles and tendons, including the tenoperiosteal junction where the tendons attach themselves to bone, the cartilaginous junctions between the vertebral bodies referred to as the discs, and fascia, the connective tissue commonly occurring in dense sheets which envelope the muscular compartments of the body.

It is crucial to the effectiveness of treatment that the cause of the problem is assessed in as much detail as possible. We think of manipulation as directed to joints. But apart from the cartilage and bone which make up the articulation, it is the pain-sensitive soft tissues, such as the ligaments, joint capsule, fat pads, and even blood vessels, which are moved, stretched and twisted. Pain and dysfunction due to muscle weakness or postural stress, for example, must be treated in the main by specific muscle re-education and postural re-alignment, and all the manipulation available will not correct those. A torn ligament, likewise, though presenting with painfully restricted joint movement, requires specific treatment directed to the ligament. Hence specific faults generally require specific treatment, and certainly manipulation directed to the joint as though it were the primary fault will in these cases meet with little success.

Before considering what conditions benefit from manipulative procedures, we must discuss the contraindications to such treatment.

Contraindications

Disease processes and injuries which affect bone and joint structures and weaken them making them especially vulnerable to stress are contraindications to all forceful manipulative procedures. In addition the use of certain drugs such as steroids and anticoagulants precludes any vigorous passive treatment.

The well-trained manipulator who works with the full knowledge of the patient's medical condition knows clearly those situations in which manipulative thrust techniques are absolutely contraindicated and those where even mobilisation is barred. He or she is also aware of conditions in which care must be exercised regarding the choice of specific techniques used and the degree of vigour which may or may not be employed. The first rule of manipulative treatment (as with all therapy) is 'do no harm', and the responsible operator always errs on the side of caution. When there is any doubt regarding the suitability of any procedure in a given situation, it is not employed.

It is the prerogative solely of the patient's doctor to diagnose the medical condition, referring the patient, as seen fit, for assessment and treatment by another properly trained professional. The referring doctor will have identified any pathology which is an absolute bar to manipulative treatment and any which requires caution.

We can list the situations in which spinal manipulation (i.e. the technique using rapid, short-amplitude thrust) is contraindicated.

1. Malignant disease of the bone or soft tissues.
2. Bone disease such as osteomyelitis, osteoporosis (of whatever cause), tuberculosis.
3. Spinal cord compression.
4. Cauda equina compression.
5. Recent fractures.
6. Vertebrobasilar insufficiency.
7. Inflammatory arthritis such as rheumatoid arthritis and ankylosing spondylitis.
8. Bony or ligamentous instability of whatever cause, e.g.

spondylolisthesis, fractures, craniocervical and lumbosacral anomalies.

9. Severe degenerative changes and long-standing spinal deformity.

10. Severe nerve root irritation or compression.

11. Pregnancy—generally all vigorous procedures to the lower thoracic and lumbar spine are to be avoided after the third month.

12. Pain of unknown origin.

13. Recent whiplash trauma to the neck.

14. Anticoagulant therapy and current or recent steroid therapy.

15. Certain psychological states where there is clear evidence the patient has developed an obsessional dependence on 'having their spine clicked back'.

A number of these conditions also preclude the use of mobilisation techniques.

Furthermore, there are situations in which particular care needs to be exercised, as with the following.

1. Severe pain, particularly if it is easily stirred and takes some time to settle.

2. Acute nerve root pain.

3. If spinal movements and/or palpation reproduce distally referred symptoms.

4. Worsening signs and symptoms such as those due to increasing nerve root compression.

Of the conditions listed as contraindications to manipulation, a number may safely be treated with mobilisation techniques provided that specific safeguards are observed. For example, the patient with known vertebral artery disease may gain great relief from the pain arising from co-existent cervical problems if treated by carefully graded mobilisation techniques. Obviously rotational movements which reproduce their dizziness will be totally avoided. But gentle traction and localised accessory movements are safe and acceptable, provided they do not aggravate the dizziness.

As another example, the patient diagnosed as having spondylolisthesis and having pain as a result of the vertebral slip frequently is afforded great relief by the use of judicious passive mobilisation. The use of any pressure techniques applied with vigour is, of course, excluded.

What, then, is suitable for treatment by manipulative procedures? Broadly, any tissue damage to the musculoskeletal structures arising from degenerative change or trauma. For the most part it is pain and abnormal inert tissue resistance which are the factors actually treated, whatever the condition which has caused them. The variety of benign peripheral and spinal joint problems for which patients may seek relief is extensive, but the majority are characterised by painfully limited movement and hence some restriction of function. Some patients seek help to loosen a stiff joint where there is little or no pain. For example, a case might be that of a long-standing shoulder capsulitis where the patient has been left with a very restricted range of joint motion or a stiff neck which prevents him turning his head to reverse the car as he could only a few weeks previously. By contrast, other patients present with severe pain, perhaps even at rest. It is their pain which dominates and prevents or restricts movement. Inert tissue resistance and stiffness are not factors, but only the disabling pain for which the patient seeks relief. An example of such a situation would be the case of someone with an acute, severe sciatica preventing them sitting and causing some misery when they attempt to stand and walk a short distance. It is the severity of the symptoms and their highly unpleasant nature for which help is sought.

While manipulative procedures will usually prove helpful in each of these cases, the techniques employed and the way in which they are carried out will be very different in the case of the severely painful compared with the severely stiff where there is little pain. We will discuss this more fully when we come to consider treatment.

Diagnosis, pathology and manipulation

Cyriax (1978), a great pioneer in the development of the treatment of musculoskeletal disorders, emphasises the paramount importance of a comprehensive and systematic examination and assessment of the moving parts of the body to make a precise diagnosis. Diagnosis is the *sine qua non* of manipulation. Provided it has been possible to make a clear-cut diagnosis of a patient's musculoskeletal problem, then this will accompany the request from the referring doctor for assessment and treatment. However, the exact cause may be unclear even though it is recognised as being a benign, mechanical one. In those cases the referral may simply state, for example, 'low back pain' or 'backache and sciatica' or 'painful, stiff shoulder' etc.

It may be that the diagnosis and the pathology implied by it come within the category which requires extra care and caution. This will be observed in these cases. Certain diagnoses, as we have seen, contraindicate the use of high-velocity thrust techniques but do not preclude the use of carefully controlled mobilisation.

A few diagnoses actually dictate precisely what specific technique should be used. As an example, nerve root irritation or compression arising from the cervical spine and giving severe and highly reactive symptoms into the upper limb should only ever be treated initially by gentle sustained cervical traction. Similarly, the patient suffering from a minor locking incident of the knee due to a meniscal tear may respond to a very specific manipulative procedure to free the mechanical block to movement arising from this internal derangement. The number of such instances when the diagnosis and pathology specifically dictate what technique must be used initially is small, however, when considered alongside the majority of musculoskeletal problems where the precise mechanisms causing the signs and symptoms are not absolutely clear.

The case of the painful stiff neck is a good example. Many such patients are x-rayed and seen to have cervical spondylosis (i.e. cervical disc degeneration). They may also have cervical arthrosis affecting the synovial apophyseal joints and the upper cervical articulations, particularly between the axis and the atlas. Now, disc degeneration is a normal process of ageing and one that eventually overtakes everybody's spine to some extent. That is not so in the case of apophyseal arthrosis which seems to occur less commonly. But the fact remains that the ubiquitous cervical spondylosis or spondylarthrosis may present clinically in a whole variety of ways, ranging from a patient with a mildly aching and slightly stiff neck to someone with a truly agonising and unpleasant pain radiating from the neck to the shoulder, arm and hand, accompanied by pins and needles, numbness and neurological changes. Both may be diagnosed as due to 'cervical spondylosis'. The treatment approaches in the two cases are entirely different. The diagnosis as such gives no indication of the precise treatment techniques to be used; it is the particular combination of signs and symptoms, in addition to certain other factors, that guides the treatment. Obviously an understanding of the nature of the problem conveyed by the diagnostic label 'spondylosis' is essential, but this more clearly defines certain boundaries within which the manipulator works rather than indicating precisely what must be done. It is certainly feasible that a number of different manipulators employing differing techniques may each provide relief to the patient with a particular type of stiff neck. They each achieve this in their own way for a variety of reasons, but the principal one is likely to be that they understand how to handle joint problems with the appropriate degree and type of movement. Each does skilfully to the painful stiff joints what is required to restore function so that they move painlessly, even though they do it employing differing techniques. This simple truth is often forgotten or ignored by some who consider themselves in possession of the precise kind of manipulative skills which best alleviate the multitude of ills which the joints of the human frame are prone to suffer.

The effects of manipulative procedures

When we discuss the effects upon the body of the various passive movement procedures, we are in danger of confusing our observations of what results from their use and how we think it may have been achieved. To guide our thinking on this matter Maitland (1977) has proposed a 'two-compartment' approach to rationalise the information we have. Firstly, there is the compartment in which we accumulate information about anatomy, biomechanics, pathology and diagnosis etc. The second compartment contains the history, signs and symptoms of any particular patient we have examined.

It is natural when discussing manipulative procedures to want to rationalise what happens during and after treatment by relating any changes in the second compartment directly to alterations in the first. However, while the effects of manipulation upon the patient's symptoms and signs can be observed and can be reported by the patient, it is speculative to attempt to describe how exactly those effects have been achieved. In other words, we cannot say precisely in any given case how we have gained an improvement in the signs and symptoms but only that we have done so.

Therefore the short answer to the question 'How and why

does manipulation work?' must, in all honesty be that we do not as yet know for certain. However, it is possible to hypothesise using the considerable volume of information now available and growing steadily relating to joint and soft tissue neurology, pathology, biomechanics and pain studies.

First, we should state that the basic effects we wish to achieve in terms of the signs and symptoms are as follows.

1. To decrease pain and other symptoms.
2. To improve mobility of the joints and soft tissues.
3. To decrease muscle spasm.

The mechanism whereby these effects are achieved by treatment would probably be one or more of the following.

1. An alteration in the bias of sensory input from the joints and soft tissues by an increase in the stimulation of the mechano-receptors located within them.

2. The prevention or limitation of the formation of inelastic scar tissue and the restoration of extensibility to the soft tissues.

3. The improvement of tissue fluid exchange.

4. The psychological effects of being carefully assessed and treated sympathetically.

These two lists are summaries of the two-compartment way of thinking about the subject mentioned earlier.

It is useful when discussing the possible ways that manipulation achieves its effects to keep in mind the cycle of events, aptly named a 'vicious circle', which is invariably encountered when the patient is taken for treatment (Fig. 2.9).

1. *Stimulation of articular mechanoreceptors and its effects upon pain.* It is only relatively recently, since the mid-1960s, that details of the morphology and precise function of the articular receptors have been known (Wyke, 1967). It represented an exciting breakthrough in knowledge for those concerned with the treatment of musculoskeletal pain and dysfunction, and in particular for manipulative therapists, since it provided evidence to demonstrate conclusively the mode of response to specific receptors (types I, II, III and IV) in joint structures to a wide spectrum of mechanical and nociceptive stimuli.

Types I, II and III are mechanoreceptors. Type III receptors are absent from the spinal joints (Wyke, 1981) but are present in the ligaments of peripheral joints. Type I articular receptors are located in the fibrous capsule of the spinal apophyseal joints.

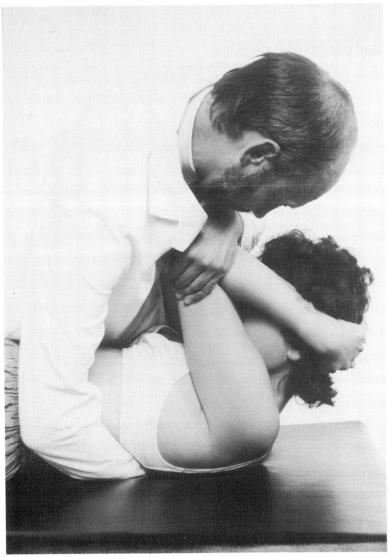

Fig. 2.9 *A thoracic manipulation localised by the underneath hand to a specific level. The force is transmitted via the operator's sternum and through the patient's arms. A localised central thoracic ache, which is neither severe nor irritable, and has failed to respond completely to mobilisation procedures, is often improved by such a procedure.*

Type II receptors can be found in the deeper layers of the capsules and in the articular fat pads. Type IV are nociceptive receptors found in the ligaments and fibrous capsules of the spinal joints, in the walls of articular blood vessels and in articular fat pads. Unlike the mechanoreceptor system, the articular nociceptive system is, under normal circumstances, completely inactive, and only becomes active when levels of mechanical stress become excessive or when chemical irritants accumulate in the tissues.

Coincidentally there was, around the same time that these receptors were described, the publication of a new theory on pain mechanisms by Melzack and Wall (1965). It took as one of its central themes the modulation of nociceptive afferent input in the spinal cord by the continual afferent barrage from mechanoreceptors. In spite of the modifications to the theory over the last two decades, this central idea has held firm and is of fundamental importance in any account seeking to show how manipulation achieves its effects. Stated briefly, one function of the mechanoreceptor system is pain suppression. When the nociceptive system is activated for any reason, the transmission of these impulses through the central nervous system will vary according to the degree of mechanoreceptor stimulation and impulse transmission occurring at the same time. The greater the level of mechanoreceptor activity, the greater the effect of pain suppression.

Consequently, as Professor Wyke (1979a and b) suggests, passive manipulation of, or the application of traction through, limb and spinal joints has many reflex and perceptual consequences. These include the relief of pain as a result of the presynaptic inhibition of pain impulses through the synapses in the basal spinal nucleus via the mechanoreceptor stimulation that is inevitably associated with all manipulative procedures. The well-trained manipulative therapist can operate this neurological mechanism with a high degree of refinement. In other words, a large part of the total effect of manipulation is achieved by modulating nociceptive and sensory input from the periphery by gaining maximal inhibitory effects from the stimulation of the mechanoreceptors located in skin fascia, muscle, tendons, ligaments, joint capsules etc. By this mechanism it is possible to break into, and thereby begin to break down, the 'vicious circle' of pain and restricted movement.

2. *Prevention of the formation of disorganised and inelastic scar tissue and the loss of extensibility in the soft tissues.* It is a fact of pathology that either by a slow process of degenerative change or as a result of sudden or repeated trauma, fibrous scar tissue is laid down within the musculoskeletal tissues. While little can be done in practice to prevent this natural healing reaction from occurring, a knowledge of the events and their time-scale helps prevent or minimise the less desirable effects of the process. The major undesirable effect of scarring within the tissues of the spinal or peripheral joints is that if it is not subjected to repeat stress at the right time, the fibres within it which give it strength will organise themselves haphazardly into a disorganised meshwork (Evans, 1980). Such an arrangement produces a weak and inextensible scar. In contrast, scar tissue which is stressed to an appropriate degree at the right stage will form within the fibres running parallel to the normal stress lines of the tissue and, with repeated movement, a mobile scar will be formed which does not restrict movement. One way of achieving some of the healthy stress upon such tissue is by manipulative techniques which utilise repeated careful stretching movements, though of course such procedures will only achieve maximal benefit if followed up by appropriate and oft-repeated movement by the patient.

The same rationale applies in the case of a spinal nerve root which is in the process of becoming adherent to the surrounding tissues, within or beyond the intervertebral foramen. Inflammation and degenerative change occurring in these tissues diminish the mobility of the nerve, which normally moves to a limited but appreciable extent during trunk and limb movements (Breig and Marions, 1963). A traumatised nerve which has become adherent in this way may be the source of chronic referred limb pain (Fahrni, 1966), and quite apart from joint manipulation, there remains the effect in such cases of 'mobilising' the nerve within the intervertebral foramen. Particular techniques are used to achieve this effect (Fig. 2.10).

3. *Improvement of tissue-fluid exchange.* The repeated functional movement of joints and their associated tissues and the contraction and relaxation of the muscles which move them during everyday activities promote the normal flow of blood and lymph by a pumping and 'milking' effect. The normal nutrition and health of tissues such as cartilage and muscle as

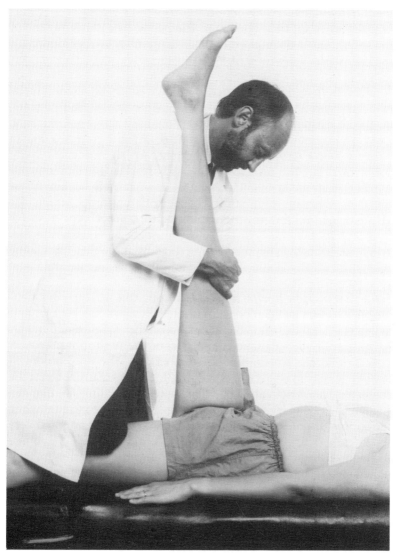

Fig 2.10 Straight leg raising technique to mobilise the pain-sensitive structures in the intervertebral canal. This treatment technique is only ever used in the presence of chronic, non-irritable symptoms when it has been estimated that some or all of the symptoms are arising from a lack of mobility between the nerve root and surrounding structures.

well as collagenous structures are probably, in part, due to such regular movement. The action of stretching which occurs naturally throughout the spine and the peripheral joints as part of the individual's normal activities maintains the extensibility of the musculoskeletal structures, especially the collagenous tissues.

When pain and joint restriction reduces such movement, often in a very masked way and for a considerable period of time, normal healthy tissue-fluid interchange is impaired (Grieve, 1981). Muscles maintained in a state of chronic guarding spasm become weak from disuse. The regular rhythmic pumping action around the affected joints is lost. The normal sensory barrage from the joint and its soft tissues is depleted. This will be the case whether it is spinal or peripheral joints which are affected. Manipulation, by helping restore movement, restores normal biomechanical forces to the muscles, collagenous tissues and local blood vessels and lymphatics. By these measures some part of its effects upon pain and mobility may be mediated.

4. *Psychological effects.* All manipulative therapy by definition involves close physical contact between the patient and operator, and the skilful and sympathetic handling of tense, painful and aching tissues. Apart from the neurophysiological effects related to manipulative therapy, the psychological benefit which may accrue from this form of treatment may be considerable. The value of 'therapeutic handling' is demonstrated every day by patients who register enormous relief when the source of their problem is found, discussed and handled very specifically and with due care. The remark 'I've longed for someone to find that spot for so long and do something about it', is satisfying to both patient and manipulator alike and when it is followed up with a demonstrable change in the patient's signs and symptoms, it helps establish a bond of trust and a spur to recovery.

How much of this effect can be ascribed to 'placebo response' is not possible to say. It is generally believed that some 20–30% of the improvement noted in any trial is due to the placebo effect, and presumably manipulation is no exception. It is still not known what the mechanisms are which underly this aspect of the total response to treatment.

On occasions a patient may appear to be developing a psychological dependence upon being manipulated. If treatment is merely reinforcing ideas of physical dysfunction when the valid testing of signs and symptoms does not bear this out, then such treatment should be reconsidered and the patient referred back to his or her doctor. We should always bear in mind that what a patient's pain and disability mean to him may differ greatly from what they mean to us. However, the limitations of manipulation must be acknowledged.

Manipulation of the disc versus the apophyseal joints

There are two further mechanisms we need to mention which in some cases are thought to be responsible for part of the response to manipulative treatment. The first concerns the phenomenon of acute joint locking and impaction of a joint meniscoid. The second concerns the effect of manipulation upon a lesion of an intervertebral disc.

The typical spinal articular triad consisting of an intervertebral disc and two apophyseal joints is the basic unit referred to when we speak of manipulating the spinal joints. It would be misguided to imagine that manipulative techniques such as those using spinal rotation or side flexion or traction can ever exclusively influence either the disc or the apophyseal joints. However, there are techniques which from clinical experience are presumed to have a greater effect when used for treating a patient suffering from a disc lesion, and there are others which appear to have greater effect where the primary fault is thought to lie within the apophyseal joints.

A subject still likely to cause acrimonious and heated discussion after many years concerns whether in manipulation it is the disc or apophyseal joints which are principally affected. Since Mixter and Barr in 1934 first implicated the disc as a cause of back and lower limb pain, there developed a tendency to become fixated by the disc as though it were the source of all the ills that befall the back. It has been argued that as a result, back pain research was held back for 40 years. The investigations of Mooney and Robertson (1976) established that the apophyseal or facet joints of the lumbar spine may equally be the source of back pain and sciatica.

The phenomenon of acute apophyseal joint locking is interesting in this respect. We know that the spinal apophyseal joints contain synovial meniscoids which project from the joint capsule into the joint cavity. Their function appears to be to increase the congruence of articular surfaces. Many manipulators have described the situation regularly seen of a patient who presents with acute spinal pain which on examination appears related to an acutely locked apophyseal joint and does not have the features of an acute disc problem. The explanation usually advanced is that a sudden unguarded movement has resulted in the joint meniscoid behaving like an intra-articular loose body interposed between the joint surfaces so as suddenly to distort the normal joint mechanics. As a result the patient is seized by a severe localised pain and violent reflex spasm. The patient is then fixed, in the case of the neck, with an asymmetrical neck posture or, in the lumbar spine, with an acute scoliotic shift. Similar pain and deformity may accompany a disc lesion but the onset, response to movement and pattern of recovery are quite different.

Acute joint locking in the cervical spine responds well to mobilisation, and very rapidly to a skilful manipulative thrust technique. The explanation for the rapid response might be that the joint is quickly gapped to free the impacted meniscoid, thereby releasing the intense spasm and thus 'unlocking' the joint. Most experts agree that the joint sound of cracking or popping which usually accompanies a manipulation is the result of a sudden gapping of the apophyseal joint in the same way that the joints of the fingers can be made to crack. In the case of the lumbar spine, the response is not usually as rapid.

Secondly there is the question of to what extent and in what way manipulation affects the disc. The universal language of the disc spoken by back sufferers has become a parody of the truth. 'Disc trouble', 'slipped disc', 'collapsed or worn out discs' or the dreaded 'crumbling spine' are discussed with great conviction and often resignation by sufferers. Only that most terrible of pronouncements 'arthritis of the spine' implies, perhaps in a way too subtle for the patient to understand, that the trouble is not primarily in the discs but in the apophyseal joints.

We need to be constantly reminded, and to remind our patients, that disc degeneration, even to the extent of prolapse, is not necessarily a painful process. The biochemical changes which parallel the biomechanical disturbances in the disc are a normal process of ageing. Spondylosis is common to us all.

The precise mechanisms whereby signs and symptoms are improved by manipulation are probably complex. For anyone to insist that they are related merely to repositioning the pulposus or parts of the annulus seems very naive in the light of our present state of knowledge. Nonetheless, it is a common experience that the techniques of traction and of regional rotation, for example, do frequently result in great benefit in cases which appear related to disc disorders. Exactly why this is so is a mystery.

Examination and assessment

No treatment, and particularly that in which manipulation technique is to be included, should ever be commenced without an appropriate and thorough examination having first been carried out by the person undertaking that treatment. Such an examination can never supplant that done by the referring doctor, but is meant to supplement it. Indeed, no logical treatment can ever be planned nor the response to it assessed until a thorough picture of the presenting signs and symptoms has been elicited, following the familiar format of 'listening, looking, testing, and feeling'.

One expert, writing of the examination preceding spinal manipulation, made the following point (Grieve, 1975): '. . . the vitally important therapist's examination is less of a diagnostic sorting procedure than an "indications" examination concerned solely with the manner in which a joint problem is manifesting itself, and with localisation of the vertebral segment(s) involved.' Exactly the same could, of course, be said of the examination of the non-spinal joints. But since manipulative treatment is associated in most people's minds with spinal problems and must take into account particular considerations of the vascularity and neurology of those regions, the points made will relate to examination and assessment of the cervical, thoracic or lumbar spine.

The subjective section of the examination will elicit the following.

1. The problem complained of, i.e. pain, stiffness, weakness, cannot work, cannot play sport, etc.
2. The precise areas of the pain and their severity, any paraesthesia and any reduced or absent sensation.
3. The type of pain, e.g. burning, throbbing, shooting, stabbing.

4. The behaviour of the different areas of pain over a 24-hour period, related to activities (such as walking, running, lifting, carrying) and postures (sitting, lying, standing). Particular attention is paid to severe night pain.

5. The history of the onset, e.g. related to a particular trauma or slow and insidious.

6. The past history, to elicit previous episodes, any pattern of development and previous treatments and their effect.

7. Points which alert the therapist to the possibility of a condition having developed which necessitates the patient being referred back to the doctor. For example, with lumbar problems, the development of retention and/or 'saddle' anaesthesia as a result of involvement of the cauda equina, or the presence of symptoms of spinal cord involvement at the cervical or thoracic levels, or sudden unexplained weight loss.

8. Details of relevant medical history and medication, e.g. diabetes, anticoagulant or steroid therapy.

Before the objective part of the examination is undertaken—literally before one places hands on the patient—it is vital to pause and consider the information elicited so far. This process of assessment, trying to make meaning of what has been gathered, will direct the remainder of the examination. While examination and assessment are two words often used interchangeably, they do not mean the same thing. It is one thing to be able to examine well but another to interpret what all the information means. As already stated, the manipulative physiotherapist's examination is not the primary diagnostic sorting procedure but more an 'indications' examination, and therefore it is the following aspects which need particularly to be decided at this point.

1. *Which structures must be tested as possibly contributing to the problem?* For example, a patient sent with a diagnosis of 'cervical spondylosis' may simply have localised unilateral neck pain with a slight restriction of movement and little else. On the other hand, the patient may present with more severe pain, a gross restriction of movement, weakness of the muscles of the shoulder girdle, neurological deficit from nerve root irritation or compression and a tight sore shoulder joint, apparently related to the chronic cervical problem. Tests which will incriminate or exclude structures over which the symptoms spread will need to be used. If muscle weakness and shoulder joint restriction are

found to be contributing to the problem, they will need to be included for treatment at some point.

2. *Are the symptoms severe?* Severity is conveyed by the degree to which the problem restricts the individual's activities. A severely stiff and painful lumbar spine, for example, may seriously affect the ability to carry on with a particular occupation or may interfere markedly with sleeping. Severe symptoms will need to be examined with great care.

3. *Is the condition irritable?* Irritability is defined by three factors: the ease with which symptoms are provoked, the intensity of those symptoms, and the time taken for them to settle following the provoking activity. Irritability must be determined before any active or passive procedures or treatment are undertaken, lest the patient's pain is unnecessarily stirred.

4. *What is the nature of the problem?* The nature of the problem has a number of aspects upon which not only the detail of the objective examination will depend but also to some extent the treatment. Two aspects may be mentioned.

(a) Serious pathology. While it is assumed that the serious disease processes which were referred to earlier as 'contraindications' have been excluded at the time of the doctor's examination, the possibility of the manifestation of such pathology during the time the patient is overseen by the physiotherapist is always kept in mind.

(b) The source of symptoms. Special consideration needs to be given as to whether the problem is, for example, primarily of the disc or of the apophyseal structures and whether the nerve root is involved and how. In this latter case the involvement of the nerve root may manifest itself as a chronic nerve root ache or, alternatively, an acute and highly irritable pain. The handling of the patient's tissues and the extent to which they are encouraged, for example, to move further during movement testing will pay due regard to all these factors. As another example, if dizziness is complained of, then the objective examination must explore this symptom in some detail so that its source, particularly if seeming to come from vertebral artery problems, can be clarified with the doctor.

The objective section of the examination will elicit the following.

1. The presence of factors which may possibly be contributing to the present problem. Examples include a short leg, poor posture, weakness of the abdominal muscles.

2. The movements that are limited and by how much and what limits them—pain, spasm or resistance.

3. Details of postural spinal deformities and whether they relate to the present episode. An example might be a lumbar scoliosis shifting the upper trunk away from or towards the painful side.

4. The presence of neurological deficit. Power, sensation and reflexes will all be tested as a routine part of the examination, particularly where pain radiates beyond the proximal joint, i.e. shoulder or hip.

5. Involvement of the pain-sensitive structures of the intervertebral canal. The straight leg raising and prone knee flexion and passive neck flexion tests will demonstrate abnormalities of dural tension and these will influence treatment and may be used to assess the efficacy of that treatment.

6. Factors which aggravate dizziness if this is complained of by the patient with a cervical problem.

7. Palpable differences in texture and in passive physiological and passive accessory intervertebral movements. This last section of the examination, palpation, is arguably the most informative and, provided no other part of the examination is omitted, skilful and meticulous palpation will help tie together all the other examination findings.

The overall aim of the objective examination is to reproduce the patient's symptoms or to aggravate them, *provided the severity, irritability and the nature of the problem permit this to be done.* The specific tests and palpation which do this are highlighted in the examination by asterisking them so that significant objective as well as subjective findings are assessed continuously to guide the treatment. When symptoms are severe, and particularly if irritable, all testing thought likely to exacerbate them is avoided, in exactly the same way as manipulative techniques judged likely to aggravate the signs and symptoms are not used.

It is the ability to monitor and interpret changes, sometimes subtle, in the many aspects of the signs and symptoms that make up one particular patient's problem, which is the key to manipulative therapy. Finely tuned assessment is the secret of the effective manipulator and not an ever-increasing store of techniques. The precise level of the spine to be treated, the type of technique used and its gentleness or vigour, the modifications, additions and subtractions to what is done are all aspects of assessment upon which the degree of success will depend. In turn all of these aspects hinge upon the abilities of the therapist as a communicator. Details of the subtle and involved process that go to make up that skill would require another chapter!

Treatment

The use of manipulative techniques is related directly to the examination findings and the assessment of those findings. Moreover, mobilisation and manipulation are chosen from a variety of different treatment techniques which the physiotherapist may choose to employ. Eventually, following due assessment, they may be used in combination with such processes as corrective exercise to enhance mobility or restore good muscle tone, postural correction and advice, or temporary splinting and supports such as a cervical collar or a lumbar corset. Manipulative therapy is not a panacea for every mechanical musculoskeletal ailment. Skilfully used, however, it will play a valuable part (and often the most important) in the overall management of the condition. Sometimes it will do so with quite dramatic effect and it is the retelling of these sudden 'cures' by one patient to another or to their doctor or by one therapist to another which has generated the myth that manipulation is a 'hole in one' curative procedure. Like most myths it is powerful, and in this instance may do considerable harm by misleading patients and doctors as to what they should expect and in making the less experienced practitioners of the art feel a failure if they do not regularly come up with such rapid successes. Every able manipulative therapist has these successes, but invariably they can be predicted. Most spinal and peripheral joint problems can be divided into those which will give a quick response and those which will take longer and even perhaps require protracted treatment—irrespective of how good the therapist is. The distinction is related to the nature of the problem and that involves the type, extent and the stage of the pathology at the time the patient is seen.

Treatment is also related not only to the relief of symptoms and signs but to advising the patient how best to avoid further episodes of pain and disablement. A knowledge of the prognosis related to various spinal syndromes is essential, therefore, in order that the manipulative therapist can give the patient realistic advice. Lumbar discogenic problems, for example, are prone to recur if the patient does not regain and maintain a good painless range of lumbar extension and flexion, habitually sits in chairs and cars with a sagging flexed posture of the lumbar spine, spends prolonged periods in sustained flexion, either while seated (as when driving) or standing, and lifts incorrectly.

When deciding the details of manipulative technique to be used, one of the principal guiding factors is whether the treatment is initially to be for pain or for inert tissue resistance and stiffness. Passive mobilisation procedures to treat pain which is severe and limits movement are carefully controlled so that they are carried out without provoking symptoms. They therefore are applied in the early part of the available range of movement, whether it be accessory or passive physiological movement. When pain is not severe nor irritable and does not limit movement markedly, the techniques used may be applied further into the range. Eventually it may be necessary to work into the pain, when this is permissible, to clear the symptoms and signs.

If restriction of movement is due to the resistance imposed by changes in the various inert soft tissues, then the techniques used will generally be applied up to and at the point of restriction, assuming that pain and muscle spasm are minimal.

A number of other factors guide the choice of technique and how it is performed. For example, in the cervical spine, if rotation is to be used, it is carried out towards the painless direction. If an acute joint locking is manipulated, a procedure is used which safely and painlessly opens the joint with great speed. There are factors which guide the manipulative therapist in selecting techniques and there is an order of efficacy to guide further the order in which they are employed.

One important guiding principle is that the force used is the minimal possible to achieve a reasonable result, and it is carefully controlled and graded. If the situation exists when a manipulative thrust technique is judged necessary, it is because it has been preceded by gentler techniques which have failed to achieve the degree of progress expected. In spite of having been applied with suitable vigour at the point of the limit in the reduced range of joint movement, mobilisations in this case will have ceased to have further effect. A manipulation may achieve the final improvement. On the other hand, mobilisation procedures may be continued after manipulation and frequently in these circumstances then achieve further improvement.

A manipulative thrust technique is used when the pain felt by the patient is a local one and only spreads locally. This is invariably related to an abnormally tight vertebral mobility segment which has been localised by passive testing. A hypermobile joint or spinal mobility segment is never manipulated, nor does a manipulation ever push through spasm.

Response to treatment

During a course of treatment it is more relevant first to ask the patient 'How have you been?' than to enquire 'How are you?' The response of the patient's symptoms to the treatment and alterations in their signs shown on testing are the factors by which progress is assessed and upon which the next treatment is planned. While there is usually a degree of immediate response to manipulative procedures and this response may be great or small, it is the behaviour of the symptoms between treatments which is the main factor we seek to influence. The manipulative therapist needs to know three things at the commencement of reassessment.

How were you in the few hours following treatment?
How have your symptoms been since the treatment and up to now?
How are your symptoms now?

Treatment may result in the patient being:
  better
  worse
  same
and it is essential before further procedures are carried out that this is clarified for all the patient's symptoms. For example, the patient who has complained of neck pain with some radiating pain into the upper arm may say that the arm pain is less noticeable. At the same time he may say his neck felt more sore for a

few hours following treatment. Additionally, he may have gained some range of movement in his neck compared with the last treatment, and may have slept better.

These points all show a good response to treatment. The soreness complained of is treatment soreness and not an exacerbation of the symptoms. The two must be clearly separated. Treatment soreness should not last more than about a day. It usually follows the treatment of joint stiffness where techniques have been used up to and at the end of the point of limitation in the range of movement. Similarly, the use of a manipulative thrust technique will usually cause some soreness for about a day.

A report by the patient that the symptoms have been worse since the last treatment must be explored carefully. They may be worse for a number of reasons. Assuming that the treatment chosen and the way it was carried out were suitable, two possibilities need to be considered.

1. The patient felt much better and so went off and did something he should not have done and made the condition worse.

2. The condition happens to be worse because its nature is that there are good and bad days and this happens to be a bad day.

Whichever the reason, it can only be ascertained by careful questioning. It is not uncommon for patients to exacerbate their pain because they feel greatly improved. They therefore imagine it is safe to dig the garden, carry heavy shopping, or go on a long car journey.

Prophylaxis is thus extremely important and it starts when the therapist not only clarifies with the patient what aggravates the condition, but also explains why it does so.

If the patient reports the symptoms are worse since last time, then the current treatment session will aim to bring the signs and symptoms back to the situation existing at the start of the last treatment session. If the treatment itself seems to have aggravated the symptoms in some way, the situation can usually be rectified by modifying the 'dosage' of treatment or altering the technique.

The rate of response

Most people wish to know how long it will take for them to

recover and be back to full normal activity. No manipulative therapist wishes to be pinned down to stating exactly how long that will be, but usually a rough time-scale can be given. It will, of course, depend largely on the nature of the problem for which the patient has sought help. Certain types of acute wry neck, for example, will require only two treatments to be pain free with a full range of neck movements. Other forms of wry neck will take about 2 or 3 weeks of treatment, initially carried out on a daily basis. The nature of the problem, and therefore the likely response to treatment, should be discussed in every case and the patient given some idea whether response will be quick or slow. If it is predicted that the response will be slow, then some discernible improvement, even though small, needs to be demonstrated at each attendance to justify continuing treatment.

The competent manipulative therapist is well able to judge whether he or she can be of help in a given situation, and should be able to do so after three or four treatments.

Recurrence of symptoms

The nature of many joint problems, particularly those of the spine, is that they are liable to recur and even grow worse. If due care is not paid by patients to their life-style, they will continue, perhaps unwittingly, to predispose themselves to further painful episodes.

Manipulative treatment aids recovery, but the maintenance of the improvement gained is the responsibility of the individual patient himself (Fig. 2.11). The most important points of prophylaxis are the maintenance of a full range of movement in all directions for the joint, and the avoidance of postures and activities which give rise to symptoms. Every patient should expect and receive careful instruction as to how best they may avoid further problems and how they may maintain full range painless movement. Manipulation may be an important factor in the patient's recovery but it is never the only one. It is often the case, for example with low back pain, that the eventual answer to a particular patient's problem in the long term is a regular regime of specific mobility exercises and meticulous attention to seated posture. The manipulative therapist is failing in his duty if this is not made very clear to the patient and pursued with sufficient emphasis.

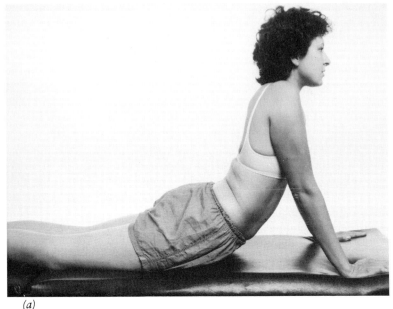

(a)

Fig. 2.11(a) *A self-mobilising procedure to regain a full lumbar exten-sion range of movement. By repeatedly raising the trunk into extension and lowering whilst maintaining the pelvis on the floor, lumbar extension is improved by a passive 'pumping' action. (b) In the presence of much stiffness, some external fixation is necessary against which the patient can work to gradually improve their range. It is im-portant that peripheral symptoms are not increased during this procedure.*

Research

The effectiveness of manipulation is not an easy thing to research. Many investigations have been undertaken, particu-larly in regard to low back pain, to compare manipulation with other forms of treatment, but a large proportion of these trials have proven very unsatisfactory for various reasons, primarily the following.

1. *The selection of patients.* In the case of low back pain, for example, a variety of mechanical causes are included. So far there is no universally accepted categorisation of the causes and mechanisms of low back pain and therefore a heterogeneous

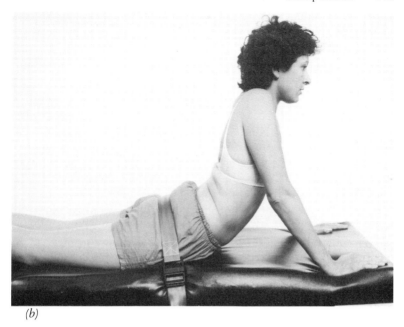

(b)

mix of pathologies and syndromes is invariably admitted into a trial. It may eventually be shown that manipulative therapy is highly effective for some conditions, less so for others or, more likely, that it achieves rapid results in certain clinical situations and slower results in others. A useful analogy can be drawn from the use of ergotamine for migraine where it has been stated that if this drug were used in a trial for headaches of a wide variety of causes, it would be shown to be ineffective. However, it is, as we know, a highly effective treatment for migraine headache.

2. *Measures for improvement.* The criteria chosen to assess progress during a trial of manipulation ultimately depend upon the patient's interpretation of pain, a subjective and highly personal factor. Even the attempts to make objective observations, such as measuring movements and the straight leg raising test used in the assessment of certain lumbar problems, do rely to a great extent on the way that pain affects the individual. The criterion of when a patient returns to work is again not a very reliable measure of real progress because individuals do so or do not do so for a varity of reasons, often unknown to those treating them. Financial and social pressures may persuade a patient to return to work even though he or she has

considerable pain, while others may not return to work even though their symptoms appear minimal.

One experienced researcher in the field stated (O'Donoghue, 1983): 'More sensitive measures of progress need to be established along with the criteria which would allow the early identification of those patients who are likely to respond to manipulation.'

3. *Personal skills of the manipulator.* If it is believed that skills of assessment and of the choice of techniques and the way they are carried out have a bearing upon the outcome of treatment, then the danger of measuring the individual skills of the operator and not 'manipulation' *per se* becomes obvious. In a trial which uses many manipulators (and they all must to obtain sufficient patient numbers in the specified time), great attempts need to be made to describe exactly what is being done under the umbrella of 'manipulation'. This is not easy, and when the choice is made too constricting as, for example, with 'one rotational manipulation each week for 3 weeks', the criticism is immediately advanced that it was not a treatment that any other manipulator would have chosen to do anyway and if it were to fail nobody would be surprised.

Double-blind and single-blind trials

The classic double-blind trial devised to test the efficacy of drugs requires that both the patients and the doctor assessing them are unaware which treatment they have received. Clearly patients are always aware whether they have or have not received 'manipulation'.

The single-blind trial, in which only the assessing doctor is unaware of the treatment, is possible but the doctor's continued lack of awareness cannot be guaranteed.

Back pain trials

A number of clinical trials on the effectiveness of various treatments, including manipulation for low back pain, have been carried out in recent years (Glover *et al.*, 1974; Evans *et al.*, 1978; Sims-Williams *et al.*, 1978). Several of them have shown that manipulation has a significant effect in benefiting patients more quickly in the short term. Several of these trials state that whatever is done does not seem to confer long-term benefit. The great problem with this conclusion is that it is based on the observations of a short course of treatment then assessed over a long follow-up period. A large proportion of low back pain sufferers have recurrent problems and many become chronic. We do not know what contribution manipulation makes to ameliorating this pattern of recurrence, and trials are needed to investigate this very large and economically important population of back sufferers.

A recent multicentre trial (Coxhead *et al.*, 1981) concerned with physiotherapy in the management of sciatic symptoms assessed four treatments: traction, exercises, manipulation, and corset. The design was factorial, thus allowing assessment of the treatments singly and in all possible combinations. Amongst the conclusions from the trial were the following.

Improvements at four weeks on the pain analogue scale tended to be greater in those receiving than not receiving a particular treatment, and in the case of manipulation the difference was statistically significant.

And, secondly:

There was good evidence that outcome at four weeks was beneficially influenced by an increasing number of types of treatment. The direct evidence for this is complemented by the clear tendency for those who have received fewer types of treatment during the trial to have further treatment in the ensuing three months.

This second conclusion is of great significance to therapists since it is common clinical practice eventually to combine treatments such as manipulation, exercise, and postural correction and advice. This is done, of course, according to specific indications and with careful assessment of the effects of each upon the changing pattern of signs and symptoms.

How to obtain manipulative treatment

A patient may choose to be treated privately or under the National Health Service. Private treatment is obtainable from physiotherapists, doctors, osteopaths and chiropractors. All osteopaths and chiropractors employ manipulative procedures in their treatments; some physiotherapists and doctors do not.

Physiotherapist manipulators

The basic physiotherapy qualification in Britain entitles the physiotherapist to become a member of the Chartered Society of Physiotherapy and thereafter to use the letters MCSP, or Member of the Chartered Society of Physiotherapy, after his or her name. Most physiotherapists, like many doctors, eventually specialise and those who choose to continue in the field of musculoskeletal disorders acquire post-registration training in the different aspects of this work, including manipulation. The Manipulation Association of Chartered Physiotherapists is a specific interest group of the Chartered Society of Physiotherapy and it maintains a regional list of members. There are, however, chartered physiotherapists who have not become members of the Manipulation Association but use manipulative procedures as part of the treatment they offer, and they are perfectly entitled to do so. Many local hospitals now have trained manipulative physiotherapists on their staff, working in close co-operation with the consultant physicians and surgeons. General practitioners frequently now send patients to the hospital anticipating that manipulative treatment may well form part of the overall management of the patient's problem. This is becoming more common with the spread of open access for GPs to refer patients directly to hospital- or community-based physiotherapists. This way patients can be treated sooner than they could hitherto when the only means of obtaining out-patient physiotherapy treatment was via a consultation with a hospital specialist. The spread of this system has increased the awareness by general practitioners of what specific treatments are available, including, of course, manipulation.

An enquiry to the superintendent physiotherapist by the doctor will clarify whether manipulative treatment is available to the patients he sends for assessment.

If a patient wishes to be treated on a private basis, then the referring doctor needs to know of local private manipulative physiotherapists to whom he can entrust his patient. The problem is that otherwise the patient, particularly if previously helped by manipulation, may take himself off to an unqualified lay manipulator. There are many individuals calling themselves physiotherapists, chiropractors or osteopaths who have not undergone the long and rigorous training demanded of those professions. Anyone can call themselves by these titles, even those who have, for example, taken a 2-week correspondence course in massage and crudely practised some manipulations from a textbook. Once again, the answer lies in communication between the referring doctor and the manipulative specialist to ascertain that the latter is properly qualified.

Osteopathic and chiropractic manipulators

Since, as stated earlier, these titles may be adopted by anyone wishing to set up a manipulative practice, it is important that a check is made of the individual's qualifications. Osteopaths who qualify to the standard of the British School of Osteopathy receive the Diploma of Osteopathy and can place DO after their names. Unfortunately, many individuals who have undertaken courses not approved by the General Council and Register of Osteopaths may also use these letters. The letters MRO, on the other hand, signify that the practitioner is a member of the Register of Osteopaths and his or her qualifications are of a sufficiently high standard to be approved by the General Council and Register of Osteopaths.

The qualification of chiropractic is Doctor of Chiropractic (DC). The British Society of Chiropractors maintains a register similar to that of the osteopaths.

Medical manipulators

The British Association of Manipulative Medicine (BAMM) was formed by a group of doctors with the aim of teaching and raising the standard of manipulative practice by doctors. The Association organises regular courses, some of them being open to physiotherapists. It is affiliated to the International Federation of Manual Medicine.

In addition, many doctors undertake training in orthopaedic medicine, a system of treatment based upon the teaching of Dr James Cyriax which includes manipulation as a major component.

References

Breig A., Marions D. (1963). Biomechanics of the lumbo-sacral nerve roots. *Acta Radiologica*; 1:1141–60.
Coxhead C. E., Inskip H., Meade T. W., North W. R. S., Troup J. D. G. (1981). Multicentre trial of physiotherapy in the management of sciatic symptoms. *Lancet*; 1:1065–8.

Cyriax J. (1978). *Textbook of Orthopaedic Medicine*, Vol. 1., 7th edn. London: Baillière Tindall.

Evans D. P., Burke M. S., Lloyd K. N., Roberts E. E., Roberts G. (1978). Lumbar spinal manipulation on trial—clinical assessment. *Rheumatology and Rehabilitation;* 17:43–53.

Evans P. (1980). The healing process at cellular level: a review. *Physiotherapy;* 66 (8):256–9.

Fahrni W. H. ((966). Observations on straight leg raising with special reference to nerve root adhesions. *Canadian Journal of Surgery;* 9:44–8.

Glover J. R., Morris J. G., Khosla T. (1974). Back pain: a randomized clinical trial of rotational manipulation of the trunk. *British Journal of Industrial Medicine;* 31:59–64.

Gray H. (1938). Sacro-iliac joint pain. *International Clinics;* 2:54–96.

Grieve G. (1975). Manipulation. *Physiotherapy;* 61 (1):11–18.

Grieve G. (1981). *Common Vertebral Joint Problems*, 1st edn. Edinburgh: Churchill Livingstone.

Janse J. (1975). History of the development of chiropractic concepts; chiropractic terminology. In *The Research Status of Spinal Manipulative Therapy*, NINCDS Monograph No. 15, pp. 25–42. Publication no. (NIH) 76–998. Washington DC: United States Department of Health Education and Welfare.

Maitland G. D. (1977). *Vertebral Manipulation*, 4th edn. London: Butterworths.

Melzack R., Wall P. D. (1965). Pain mechanisms: a new theory. *Science (New York);* 150:971–9.

Mixter W. J., Barr J. S. (1934). Rupture of the intervertebral disc with involvement of the spinal cord. *New England Journal of Medicine;* 211:210.

Mooney V., Robertson J. (1976). The facet syndrome. *Clinical Orthopaedics and Related Research;* 115:149–56.

Northup G. W. (1975). History of the development of concepts; osteopathic terminology. In *The Research Status of Spinal Manipulative Therapy*, NINCDS Monograph No. 15, pp. 43–51. Publication No. (NIH) 76–998. Washington DC: United States Department of Health Education and Welfare.

O'Donoghue C. E. (1983). Controlled trials of manipulation. *Newsletter, The Manipulation Association of Chartered Physiotherapists;* 14:1–6.

Schiotz E., Cyriax J. (1975). *Manipulation Past and Present*. London: William Heinemann Medical Books.

Sims-Williams H., Jayson M. I. V., Young S. M. S., Baddeley H., Collins E. (1978). Controlled trial of mobilisation and manipulation for patients with low back pain in general practice. *British Medical Journal;* 2:1338–40.

Wyke B. D. (1967). The neurology of joints. *Annals of the Royal College of Surgeons of England*; **41**:25.

Wyke E. D. (1979a). Articular neurology and manipulative therapy. In *Aspects of Manipulative Therapy*, pp. 67–72. Melbourne: Lincoln Institute of Health Sciences.

Wyke E. D. (1979b). Neurology of the cervical spinal joints. *Physiotherapy*; **65**(3):72–6.

Wyke E. D. (1981). The neurology of joints: a review of general principles. *The Biology of the Joint, Clinics in Rheumatic Diseases*, 7 (1), pp. 223–39. Philadelphia: W. B. Saunders.

Useful addresses

British Association of Manipulative Medicine
62 Wimpole Street
London W1M 7DY.

British School of Osteopathy
1–4 Suffolk Place
London SW1

British Chiropractors Association
5 First Avenue
Chelmsford
Essex CM1 1RX.

The Chiropractic Medical Association
51 Canford Cliffs Road
Poole
Dorset.

Anglo European Chiropractic College
13 Parkwood Road
Bournemouth
Dorset BH5 2DF.

The London College of Osteopathic Medicine
8–10 Boston Place
London NW1 6QH.

General Council and Register of Osteopaths
1–4 Suffolk Street
London SW1Y 4HG.

The Manipulation Association of Chartered Physiotherapists
c/o The Professional Consultant
The Chartered Society of Physiotherapists
14 Bedford Row
London WC1R 4ED.

The Organisation of Chartered Physiotherapists
  in Private Practice
14 Bedford Row
London WC1R 4ED.

The Institute of Orthopaedic Medicine
c/o Dr M. Hutson (Secretary)
30 Park Row
Nottingham.

The Association of Chartered Physiotherapists
  in Sports Medicine
14 Bedford Row
London WC1R 4ED.

The author would like to thank Mr Simon Brown ARPS, medical photographer at St Stephens Hospital, Fulham, for his invaluable help in preparing the illustrations.

Chapter 3

Biofeedback and meditation
D. Marcer

The purpose of this chapter is to introduce the reader to the
clinical application of biofeedback and various forms of relaxation therapy in treating stress-linked illnesses. Within the
confines of the available space this is no easy task, for both
forms of treatment are now the subject of a large and expanding
literature. To take just one example: a recent text devoted to biofeedback runs to 390 pages, lists more than 700 published
references, and describes more than 20 applications of this
method alone (Basmajian, 1983). Clearly such detailed coverage
is beyond the scope of a single chapter, especially one which also
seeks to evaluate the current status of relaxation therapy.

I have attempted to solve the problem by dealing in depth with
just two chronic conditions: essential hypertension and
headache. There are two reasons for this choice. First, both are
common conditions which place heavy demands on the health
services. Second, both have been widely treated by biofeedback
and relaxation, thus allowing some important theoretical issues
to be illustrated. In order to do so, I have prefaced each section
with a brief description of the condition under consideration.
While I believe that what I have written is accurate, it does not
pretend to be more than a very simple account. Certainly
nobody should believe that the information is sufficiently
detailed to allow them to make an accurate diagnosis; even less
to plan a course of treatment!

I have paid readers the compliment of assuming that they will
wish to judge for themselves the claims that have been made for
these forms of treatment, as well as my evaluation of them. To
this end I have outlined their theoretical bases, preferring to
describe a few seminal findings in some detail, rather than
merely listing a vast number of studies without any critical

evaluation. Finally, I have not dealt with a number of important applications of biofeedback, especially in the areas of neurology and rehabilitation. The interested reader should consult Basmajian (1983).

Introduction

Over the past century the Western industrialised world has witnessed a remarkable shift in disease patterns. Thanks largely to improvement in public health services, aided by advances in pharmacology, many communicable diseases have for all practical purposes been eradicated. At the same time, however, there has been an alarming increase in non-infectious disease. For example, the incidence of coronary heart disease has risen dramatically, and Seer (1979) has described hypertension as reaching epidemic proportions. Similarly, disorders such as chronic headache, anxiety states and gastrointestinal disturbances continue to place an ever-increasing burden on our overstretched health care resources. Because these disorders develop slowly—often throughout the sufferer's adult life—they are much more vulnerable to psychological influences. This, plus the fact that they are not caused by infection, has led many writers to speculate that they are the direct result of the stresses of modern life. As will be seen in the second half of this chapter, psychological stress is undoubtedly associated with many chronic illnesses, including a whole range of physical conditions. However, an association does not necessarily imply a cause, and the precise role played by stress in the aetiology and maintenance of physical illness is still the subject of heated, and frequently acrimonious, debate. Nevertheless, most family doctors would agree that stress is at the heart of some of the most intractable cases that they are called upon to treat. It is against the above background that there has been a re-awakening of interest in a number of techniques, all of which can loosely be described as self-control therapies. These include meditation, biofeedback, various forms of relaxation training, yoga, and hypnosis. This chapter is confined to an evaluation of the current status of the first three.

Meditation

It was only when I came to prepare this chapter that I became aware of the number of practices that now exist in the Western world under the guise of meditation or relaxation. These range from the relatively modest techniques that are associated with natural childbirth, to quasi-religious systems such as transcendental meditation (TM). Given such a diversity of practices, we are immediately faced with a problem of definition. This is especially so in the case of meditation, which dates back to pre-Christian times, and encompasses a wide range of behaviour, from ritual dancing at one extreme to tranquil relaxed states at the other. In an attempt to incorporate the elements common to all of these practices into a single definition, Shapiro (1982) has proposed that meditation refers to: 'a family of techniques which have in common a conscious attempt to focus attention in a non-analytic way and an attempt not to dwell on ruminating discursive thought'.

This definition clearly embraces those forms of meditation most commonly practised in the Western world. For example, TM requires the individual to spend two 20-minute sessions each day with eyes closed, silently repeating a specially selected Sanskrit sound, or mantra. This constant repetition of a word or phrase is to be found in many meditative practices, and as long ago as the fourteenth century Gregory of Sinai taught that the 'Jesus Prayer' should be repeated quietly, and in rhythm with the exhalation phase of breathing.

As well as differing in their methods, meditative techniques can also have quite different objectives. Thus, this chapter is devoted to their use as a therapeutic measure. However, the last thing that concerned Gregory was to develop an alternative treatment for essential hypertension or migraine! In common with all meditation occurring within a religious context, be it Christianity, Shintoism or Taoism, his purpose was to achieve union with God, or some form of 'ultimate reality'. While this metaphysical perspective poses no problems for some individuals, there will be many others, raised in the present-day climate of scientific objectivity, who find it inappropriate. In an attempt to overcome this problem, Professor Herbert Benson and his colleagues (1977) have developed what they describe as a simple, non-cultic technique, in which the subject is given the following instructions.

(a) Sit quietly in a comfortable position and close your eyes.

(b) Deeply relax all your muscles, beginning at your feet and progressing up to your face. Keep them deeply relaxed.

(c) Breathe through your nose. Become aware of your breathing. As you breathe out say the word *one* silently to yourself. For example, breath in ... out, *one*, in ... out, *one*, etc. Continue for 20 minutes. You may open your eyes to check the time, but do not use an alarm. When you finish, sit quietly for several minutes at first with closed eyes and later with opened eyes.

(d) Do not worry about whether you are successful in achieving a deep level of relaxation. Maintain a passive attitude and permit relaxation to occur at its own pace. Expect other thoughts. When these distracting thoughts occur ignore them by thinking 'Oh well' and continue to repeat 'one'. With practice the response should come with little effort. Practise the technique once or twice daily, but not within two hours after any meal, since the digestive processes seem to interfere with the subjective changes.

It is obvious that despite being separated by almost six centuries, the techniques devised by Gregory and Benson have much in common. For example, both utilise subvocalisation which is synchronised with breathing, both are passive, and, while encouraging the participant to ignore other thoughts, adopt a benign attitude should they intrude. However, though they may resemble each other methodologically, there the resemblance ends. For, as was previously noted, the follower of Gregory seeks union with God, while Benson's procedure is intended to do no more than produce a state of deep relaxation. Although this appears to be a modest objective, Benson has argued that the relaxation response is a unique physiological state, and is the common denominator which underlies virtually all meditative techniques.

The relaxation response

From the outset it has to be made clear that Benson ascribes more meaning to the term 'relaxation' than is implied in normal usage. For some readers the word might suggest an evening sitting in front of a warm fire, enjoying a glass of sherry and reading a good book. Others take their relaxation in a more active manner, such as a golfing or sailing holiday. Benson, however, is referring to an integrated hypothalamic response which 'is consistent with generalised decreased sympathetic nervous activity'. Moreover, four elements are identified as necessary to evoke this response: a quiet environment, decreased muscle tone, a repeated sound, word or phrase, and a passive attitude (Benson *et al.*, 1977, p. 442). In other words, the unique physiological effect of meditation is to attenuate activity within the sympathetic branch of the autonomic nervous system (ANS). This is an extremely important hypothesis, for it is widely acknowledged that the sympathetic nervous system (SNS) is intimately involved in our response to stress.

The autonomic nervous system

All our behaviour is controlled by either the central nervous system (CNS) or the autonomic nervous system (ANS). The CNS, which encompasses the brain and spinal cord, controls the musculoskeletal activity, while the ANS innervates the internal organs, glands, heart, lungs and smooth muscles. Traditionally, responses mediated by the ANS were thought to be of a reflex nature and outside the voluntary control of the individual, though, as we shall see later, this view was strongly challenged in the 1960s. The ANS is further divided into two systems, the sympathetic (SNS) and the parasympathetic (PNS). Although to some extent both systems are always active, the two sets of behaviour that they control tend to be incompatible. Thus, PNS activity dominates during the processes of digestion, relaxation and sleep, while the SNS controls behaviour that is preparatory to action, including what has come to be known as the fight or flight response.

The fight or flight response

When an organism is threatened with imminent danger, certain physiological changes take place due to increased SNS activity. There is an increased production of catecholamines, which leads to increased heart rate and, initially at least, raised blood pressure. Blood flow to the skeletal muscles and coronary arteries is increased at the expense of the digestive system, the activity of which is inhibited. The pupils dilate, blood sugar levels increase, and the gastrointestinal and bladder sphincters are closed. It is readily apparent that although such changes prepare the organism for action, it is action of an extreme physical nature. Within an evolutionary framework, this no doubt makes very good sense. Faced with a predator, early man would have little choice but to fight or take flight. However, such behaviour is rarely appropriate to the stresses encountered in modern society. We are no longer faced with the sabre-tooth tiger or the woolly mammoth. Instead we are called upon to deal with their modern counterparts, the uncommunicative garage mechanic, or the receptionist who has dedicated her life to preventing us from seeing the doctor.

Once we accept that the fight or flight response is inappropriate to many of the demands of living in a competitive, industrialised society, we are offered an explanation of how stress might be linked to organic illness. Faced with psychological stress rather than bodily threat, increased SNS output will no longer be dissipated by a corresponding increase in physical activity. Hence, over long periods of time, inappropriate increases in heart rate and blood pressure, along with interruption of the digestive and other metabolic processes, might well produce and exacerbate pathology in the corresponding organs. Although this is an appealing hypothesis, we need to be clear that at present it is no more than that. Moreover, like all hypotheses, it raises a number of questions. Perhaps the most crucial concerns the maintenance of the high level of SNS output that is assumed to underlie the development of organic illness. Surely, once we realise that the fight or flight response is no longer appropriate, it will disappear from our behavioural repertoire. In fact the evidence suggests otherwise. Once established, responses involving the SNS are remarkably resistant to extinction. Thus, we still experience a momentary churning in the stomach when visiting the dentist, even though at a cognitive level we know there is nothing to fear.

The stability of the SNS responses has long been known to those psychologists interested in the basic principles of learning. For example, Liddell (1934) demonstrated that classically conditioned autonomic responses in sheep long outlive their overt behavioural counterparts, often by many years. Unfortunately, the nature of the SNS is such that experimental investigation of its function involves exposing the subject to painful stimuli, usually electric shock. For ethical reasons, therefore, few studies involving human subjects have been reported. However, the limited evidence that is available suggests that in this respect at least, we are not too unlike sheep.

The preceding discussion provides enough evidence to take seriously the hypothesis that stress and organic illness are linked as a result of inappropriate SNS output. Note, however, this need not imply a causal relationship. For example, although there is little evidence that coronary heart disease is *caused* by stress, it is recognised that the condition may be exacerbated by the increase in blood pressure which stress evokes.

Meditation and stress

If, as Benson believes, the relaxation response produces decreased SNS activity, then we can begin to see how meditation might be of therapeutic value. In fact a number of laboratory investigations have shown that meditation is accompanied by lowered blood pressure, muscle tone, and skin conductance; decreased oxygen consumption and carbon dioxide elimination; slowing of the pulse; and lowered levels of lactate and catecholamines in the blood. However, it has also been demonstrated that these changes are not unique to meditation. Although this conclusion would be challenged by some researchers, the consensus is that the physiological changes that occur as a result of meditation can also be achieved by other techniques, including controlled muscular relaxation (Fenwick, 1983). Consequently, throughout the remainder of this chapter, the terms meditation and deep relaxation will be regarded as synonymous. A much more important question than whether or not meditation produces a unique physiological effect is the extent to which this effect outlasts the actual period of meditation. What the chronic hypertensive needs is something more than a technique which lowers his blood pressure twice daily for 20 minutes. To be of any lasting therapeutic value the effect must be robust enough to survive outside the tranquil confines of the treatment session. However, as this is true of any treatment, discussion will be postponed until after the final therapy to be evaluated has been outlined.

Biofeedback

The justification for using meditation as a therapeutic measure is its alleged ability to damp down the activity of the SNS. In so far as the SNS tends to act as a single unit, meditation will result in a general reduction in the behaviours under its control. The early proponents of biofeedback, on the other hand, argued that by the use of appropriate monitoring devices, an individual could learn to control specific autonomic responses. Thus, one individual might normalise his blood pressure, another regularise his heart rate, while a third would learn to increase the flow of blood to his hands. Indeed, given the appropriate feedback, virtually no physiological system would be beyond our control. Moreover, all this would be achieved by a process of directed trial-and-error learning, rather than a general damping down of the SNS.

Undoubtedly trial-and-error learning is heavily dependent upon feedback, as anyone who has tried to learn to play snooker will readily acknowledge. For only after prolonged practice do we acquire the skill to strike the cue ball so that it hits the target ball, before ending up approximately where we intended. The development of such a skill not only relies on visual feedback, but also requires kineasthetic information from the muscles and joints to tell us how hard we struck the cue ball, how tightly we were holding the cue, and the position of our feet relative to the rest of our body. Clearly, without such feedback it would be impossible to learn the smooth, coordinated movements which are the hallmark of a champion games player.

Not only is feedback crucial for learning to occur, it continues to be so if a learned skill is to be maintained. Nowhere is this more apparent than in those cases where loss of feedback occurs as a result of pathology. Many readers will be aware how quickly severe deafness disrupts the ability of the sufferer to produce rhythmical speech. Less common, but much more spectacular, are the ataxias, which arise from pathology of the nervous system and involve a loss of muscular coordination, without necessarily a loss of muscular power. Before the advent of penicillin it was possible to encounter advanced cases of *tabes dorsalis*, a disease of the dorsal column which produces a loss of proprioceptive feedback from the limbs. Thus, in order to know the position of his arms and legs, the sufferer has to rely on visual feedback alone, with results that are little short of devastating. In the dark he frequently falls over, and is unable to point in a given direction. Gait becomes exaggerated, as he walks by raising his legs excessively, looking intently downwards, and slapping his feet to the ground. This last example provides an especially powerful demonstration of the crucial part played by feedback in behaviour carried out via the musculoskeletal system. However, such behaviour is controlled by the CNS, and, as we have already seen, it is assumed that the link between stress and organic illness involves inappropriate SNS activity. What evidence is there that feedback will enable us to gain voluntary control of this behaviour?

The conditioning of autonomic responses

For many years it was widely accepted that autonomic responses could not be brought under voluntary control. However, in the 1960s the American psychologist Neal Miller and his associates published a series of papers which challenged this view. Briefly, Miller claimed that it was possible to learn to control a wide range of autonomic responses. These included heart rate, blood pressure and distribution, and the rate of flow of urine in the kidneys. Most of Miller's findings derived from experiments on rats which had been temporarily paralysed with curare, so ensuring that any change in behaviour represented true autonomic learning and was not being mediated via the musculoskeletal system. The question of mediation is one which still divides behavioural scientists concerned with the nature of the learning process. However, it need not concern us here, although we shall return to the issue when we come to evaluate the efficacy of biofeedback. For purely clinical purposes, it matters little whether the ability to control blood pressure is achieved directly as a result of autonomic conditioning or via mediating musculoskeletal activity. However, it must be stated that since the publication of Miller's earliest studies many scientists have been unable to replicate his findings. Indeed, in 1978 Miller wrote that prudence dictated that it was unwise to rely on his work on curarised animals as evidence that visceral responses could be brought under direct voluntary control. By then, however, biofeedback had become an established form of treatment. Consequently practitioners were more inclined to direct their efforts to measuring efficacy, than to become further embroiled in theoretical issues.

Methods of biofeedback

Although biofeedback frequently involves the use of complex electronic instruments, these are nothing more than measuring tools whose nature will be determined by the physiological system under review. In this chapter the discussion is confined to the four types of feedback most commonly encountered in clinical practice.

Direct feedback of blood pressure

Not surprisingly, this form of feedback was widely adopted in early attempts to teach hypertensive patients to reduce blood pressure. The actual techniques ranged from training the patient in the use of a simple mercury sphygmomanometer, to methods which rely upon quite elaborate, semi-automatic devices. However, whatever the method, they all sought to make the patient aware of any change in blood pressure.

The galvanic skin response (GSR)

Although it must be stated at the outset that the mechanisms underlying the GSR are still the subject of some debate, it is one of the most widely used indices of autonomic arousal. Its use is based upon the finding that sweat gland activity increases as a function of autonomic arousal, with a corresponding decrease in skin resistance. Biofeedback makes use of this fact by measuring changes in resistance between two electrodes fastened to the patient's fingers (Fig. 3.1). These changes are then converted to a form which can be observed directly, usually as a rise or fall in the frequency of a tone. It should be noted that changes in GSR can be brought about by a large number of extraneous factors including temperature, humidity, and precise placement of the electrodes. As it is rarely possible to control these factors within a clinical setting, intersessional differences in GSR must be interpreted with extreme caution.

Electromyogram (EMG) feedback

This particular form of feedback makes use of the fact that electrodes placed on the skin can be used to detect small changes in electrical activity which are known to occur with changes in the tension of underlying muscles. It is then a relatively simple matter to convert these electrical changes into an auditory or visual form. Two points need to be made about this particular form of feedback. First, the EMG is not an index of anxiety, tranquillity or any other mental state; it is simply a measure of muscular contraction which may or may not correlate with our state of mind. Second, electrical activity which is measured at the skin surface will not represent the output of a single muscle. For example, the label frontalis feedback is often applied to this technique when it is used in the treatment of headaches (Fig. 3.2). Although the electrodes are placed over the frontalis muscles, they are likely to detect changes in other muscles as

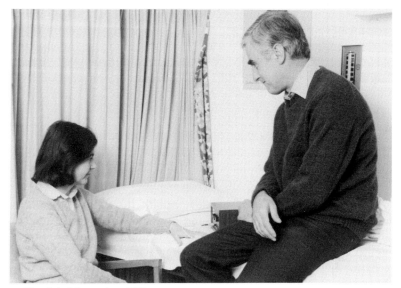

Fig. 3.1 Measuring GSR.

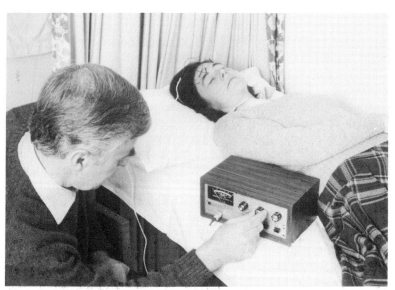

Fig. 3.2 EMG feedback training.

well, especially those of the face, jaw, and scalp. It is also worth noting here that the question of whether feedback can lead to direct conditioning of autonomic responses does not arise in this case. Clearly, EMG feedback is concerned entirely with acquiring control of the musculoskeletal system.

Temperature feedback

As the name implies, this form of feedback involves providing the patient with information about changes in body temperature. This is usually achieved by using an appropriately placed thermistor sensor which can detect changes as small as 0.001°C.

These then are the technical details of the forms of biofeedback most commonly encountered in clinical practice. However, the prospective patient is usually less interested in this sort of detail than in what will actually happen to him, whether the treatment is invasive (either physically or psychologically) and how long it is likely to last. Unfortunately, although the use of biofeedback is commonplace in the USA, it is only rarely encountered in the UK, and many NHS doctors would be unable to provide this sort of information. Certainly my own clinical colleagues are only half joking when they eye my consulting room suspiciously and enquire what exactly I get up to in there!

The first thing that should be emphasised to the prospective patient is that although the equipment might suggest otherwise, no electric shocks are involved. Many patients are understandably suspicious, and some downright terrified of any treatment which requires electrodes to be fitted, especially to their foreheads. Frontalis EMG feedback is, therefore, particularly suspect in this respect, and I have had to reassure more than one patient that he was not in fact being prescribed a course of ECT (electroconvulsive therapy). The second fear expressed by many patients is that they will 'lose control of their minds' or be hypnotised. Again this is a fear that can be easily resolved. The whole rationale of biofeedback is that although the therapist might suggest ways of attaining a relaxed state, it is the patient who controls his own behaviour.

In summary, virtually every form of feedback involves the patient in nothing more than sitting or lying comfortably, and adopting whatever strategy he finds appropriate to reach a relaxed state. Although courses of treatment may vary in length, they rarely exceed 10–15 half-hour sessions. For example, my own practice is to see a patient for eight weekly sessions, at the end of which we review his progress. If we both feel that he is deriving benefit, we usually continue for a further six sessions on a less regular basis. At the same time the patient is urged to practise daily what he has learned in the clinic, usually without the assistance of equipment.

Hypertension

Hypertension has been described as having reached epidemic proportions. In practice it is difficult to define the precise prevalence, for there is no cut-off point above which normal blood pressure suddenly becomes abnormal. Using the World Health Organisation's criterion of 160/95 mmHg, several surveys show that up to 10% of the male population in the UK are hypertensive. Of all these cases, only 10% are the result of known pathology, of which 90% involve renal disease. For the remaining 90% no cause is identifiable, and it is still a matter of debate whether this condition, essential hypertension, is a single entity with one or more causes, or a group of quite different entities, each with its own specific cause.

Stress and hypertension

Given the failure to identify an organic basis for so many cases of hypertension, it is hardly surprising that interest has focused on the part played by psychological stress in its aetiology and maintenance. For we have already seen that the body's response to stress—the fight or flight response—involves a number of physiological changes, including a temporary increase in blood pressure.

Further evidence linking stress with hypertension comes from surveys of occupational groups that are known to work under consistently high levels of psychological pressure. For example, the prevalence of hypertension is greater amongst air-traffic controllers working in areas of high traffic density than it is amongst their colleagues working under less demanding conditions. Parallel findings have been reported from animal studies, where not only is blood pressure seen to increase during periods of experimentally induced stress, but the effect persists beyond the duration of the experiment. It is possible to cite many similar examples, though as was emphasised at the very outset, none of them provides an unequivocal demonstration that stress, or any other psychological factor, is a direct cause of essential hypertension. Moreover, even if a causal relationship were to be established, it would not necessarily follow that purely psychological techniques would provide effective treatment. It is well documented that chronic essential hypertension produces structural changes in the vasculature which serve to maintain the condition. It is no more reasonable to expect that these secondary increases would respond to psychological treatment than it is to suggest that giving up smoking would cure advanced lung cancer. However, despite these qualifications, the link between hypertension and stress is well enough established to justify investigating the part that therapies based upon psychological principles might have to play in its control.

Behavioural control of hypertension

Meditation

The case for using meditation to treat hypertension rests primarily on two assumptions.

1. The stresses of modern living produce inappropriately high levels of SNS activity which are manifested in the fight or flight response.
2. By damping down the activity of the SNS, meditation produces a number of physiological changes, including a lowering of blood pressure.

The hypothesis that meditation had a clinical role gained credence when early studies suggested that individuals who regularly practised TM were less prone to a wide range of medical disorders. Unfortunately, these studies were almost invariably poorly designed, and lacking necessary controls, while the fact that many emanated from within the TM movement rendered them especially vulnerable to unintentional experimenter bias. Moreover, even if we accept the findings at their face value, they present a particularly difficult problem of interpretation. For it is highly unlikely that an individual would become a dedicated meditator without at the same time changing other aspects of his life-style, any one of which could have been responsible for the favourable outcome.

In fact subsequent research was to indicate that although meditation might have a part to play in the treatment of mild hypertension, it is a much more modest part than the early enthusiasts had hoped for. For example, Benson and his associates reported that following a programme of TM, a group of 22 untreated, borderline hypertensives exhibited a mean blood pressure of 139.5/90.8 mmHg, compared with a pre-treatment level of 146/94.6 mmHg. Although the decline of 6.5/3.8 mmHg was statistically significant, changes of this magnitude rarely have any clinical relevance. Moreover, no long-term follow-up data were provided, and there is evidence that the effects of TM on raised blood pressure can be relatively unstable. For example, Pollack *et al.* (1977) reported that 20 hypertensives undertaking TM showed small decreases in systolic pressure early in the programme, but these had disappeared at 6 months. The authors concluded that it is unlikely that TM has a direct effect on raised blood pressure. Rather less pessimistic findings were reported by Blackwell *et al.* (1976) who found that following a 12-week programme of TM, six out of seven hypertensives showed significant reductions in blood pressure, which in two cases were maintained at a 6-month follow-up. It is interesting to note that in this study patients were required to measure their own pressure up to four times daily. The preceding three studies are typical of the literature, and lead to the conclusion that when used alone meditation does not offer an alternative to conventional treatment, although small decreases in pressure do frequently occur.

Biofeedback

The earliest clinical applications of biofeedback were not, of course, intended to combat the general effects of stress, but sought to teach the patient how to gain voluntary control of a specific autonomic response. Initially it did indeed appear that continuous or intermittent feedback was all that the hypertensive needed in order to regulate his blood pressure. One of the earliest successful applications of direct feedback was reported by Miller (1972), who described how a hypertensive patient learned to lower her diastolic pressure from 97 to 76 mmHg, and at the same time ceased antihypertensive medication. Regrettably, this early success proved very difficult to repeat, and although a number of subsequent studies have reported favourable outcomes, they have been much more modest.

One study that deserves a special mention is that reported by Kristt and Engel (1975) in which four patients entered a 3-week training programme in which they learned to raise and lower blood pressure successively. This study is noteworthy because it is one of the very few to present follow-up data. These showed that 3 months after formal training ended, the mean pressure as measured at home was 144/87 mmHg, compared with a pre-training baseline of 162/94 mmHg. A further interesting aspect of this study is that throughout the follow-up period, patients were required to continue the training procedure at home, and to keep a daily record of their performance. This was one of the earliest studies to employ an element of self-management, and as we shall see in the next section, subsequent research suggests that this is a crucial aspect of behavioural treatment. Unfortunately, direct feedback and self-monitoring require elaborate equipment, and no mean level of technical competence on the part of the operator. This fact alone partly explains why relatively little effort has been made to build upon the work of Kristt and Engel. However, the biggest single factor to inhibit the development of this technique is that favourable outcomes have proved notoriously difficult to replicate. This is well illustrated by the work of Edward Blanchard, a pioneer in this particular area of biofeedback. Following early success, he subsequently reported that direct feedback training, followed by home practice, resulted in '*no* significant differential effects of treatment (compared with EMG feedback or simple relaxation) and very small treatment effects *per se*' (Blanchard, 1979).

As this brief review makes clear, although they are based upon different premises, the histories of direct feedback and meditation as they relate to hypertension have followed remarkably similar courses. In both cases early euphoria gave way to disenchantment, as it became increasingly obvious that their effects were small, and sometimes transitory. Indeed, one authority has gone so far as to suggest that meditation might simply be a placebo, which shows diminishing returns over time. Implicit in this argument is the assumption that if we were able to eliminate the placebo effect completely, then meditation would have nothing unique to contribute. Yet to suggest that a decrease in blood pressure is no more than an uncontrolled placebo effect is to concede that the vascular system is controlled, at least in part, by psychological factors. We ought not, therefore, to abandon too readily the search for a method whereby such factors can be utilised to the patient's advantage. In fact, evidence is beginning to emerge that psychological techniques, which used alone are relatively ineffective, can combine to produce quite powerful effects.

The conjoint treatment of hypertension

Throughout the 1970s a series of papers appeared in the medical journals which described how behavioural methods had been used to control hypertension. These were the work of Dr Chandra Patel, a family doctor who practises in South London. What makes Patel's work worthy of special note is that she reports decreases in blood pressure far in excess of any that have been achieved elsewhere. Because her methods have implications for behavioural control therapies in general, it is worth considering her work in some detail.

Unlike the studies discussed in the previous section, Patel combines four interrelated psychological components into a single treatment programme. The following is a summary of one such programme (Patel and North, 1975) which, apart from minor modifications, characterises the majority of her research in this area.

Seventeen hypertensive patients underwent treatment, each attending 12 ½-hour sessions, spread over a period of 6 weeks, at which they received training in biofeedback-assisted meditation. Members of a control group attended for an equal number of sessions, during which they were simply asked to relax, and received no further instructions.

Relaxation/meditation

Although Patel uses the term 'yoga' to describe this component, it is for all practical purposes identical to the method devised by Benson *et al.* in order to elicit the relaxation response (see page 111).

Biofeedback

Throughout the meditation sessions, both GSR and EMG feedback were provided, usually in that order. It is worth noting here that direct blood pressure feedback was not utilised, though patients had access to their records throughout the trial.

Practice

Not only were patients required to practise meditation for 20 minutes twice daily at home, they were also encouraged to incorporate these habits into routine activities. For example, they were told to relax at the sound of the telephone, and had a small red disc attached to their watches to remind them to relax whenever they looked at the time.

Information and motivation

Prior to the trial, patients attended meetings at which they were shown slides and films dealing with hypertension. These were designed to illustrate how emotion is related to bodily processes, the physiology of relaxation, as well as explaining the concepts of biofeedback and self-control. Furthermore, the meetings served to increase the motivation of the patients. To quote the authors: 'The rapport created between doctor and patients as well as that between patients themselves helped to strengthen the programme and ensure cooperation.'

A novel aspect of the study was that it comprised two separate phases. Thus, 5 months after the end of Phase 1, both groups re-entered the trial. However, this time their roles were reversed: the original control group underwent treatment, while the original treatment group served as controls. The data from each phase of the study are shown in Table 3.1. The findings can be summarised as follows.

1. By the end of Phase 1 the treated group had undergone a mean drop in blood pressure of 26.1/15.2 mmHg, compared with only 8.9/4.2 mmHg in the case of controls.

2. By the beginning of Phase 2 the improvement in the treated group had been maintained, even though they had received no further treatment during the 5-month interval.

3. By the end of Phase 2 the original control group was showing decreases that were almost identical to those achieved by the treated group in Phase 1.

4. The decreases were not uniform across subjects, but varied from 60/30 mmHg at one extreme, to 7/1 mmHg at the other. (The data are shown in this form for convenience. The systolic and diastolic falls did not necessarily occur in the same patient.)

5. Compared with controls, the treated patients showed smaller increases in blood pressure when subjected to experimental stress.

Table 3.1 Effects of conjoint behavioural treatment on hypertension (based on Patel and North, 1975)

		Group no.	Mean initial blood pressure (mmHg)		Mean final blood pressure (mmHg)	
			Systolic	Diastolic	Systolic	Diastolic
Phase 1	Treated	17	167.5	99.6	141.4	84.4
	Control	17	168.9	100.6	160.0	96.4
Phase 2	Treated (formerly control)	16	176.6	104.3	148.6	89.3
	Control (formerly treated)	17	148.8	87.8	146.2	86.2

Perhaps the first thing that should be said about these findings is that given the number of false dawns that have occurred over the past two decades, there is a great need for corroboration by other research groups. However, apart from relatively short baseline periods, it must be emphasised that there are no obvious methodological grounds for criticising these studies. Indeed, they represent some of the more sophisticated clinical research in this area. For example, the data shown in Table 3.1 are based upon readings taken *before* the relaxation session, and offer, therefore, a truer indication of the patient's 'real-life' blood pressure. Furthermore, they were taken by a nurse who was not aware whether the patient was undergoing treatment or acting as a control. Although not entirely compensating for the lack of a formal placebo group, the use of a cross-over design allowed some tentative conclusions to be drawn about treatment-specific effects, and in the case of the original treatment group demonstrated that the effect was relatively robust. (The provision of precise double-blind placebo control is especially problematical in studies of this nature. In the conventional drug trial it is relatively simple to ensure that neither doctor nor patient knows who is receiving the dummy pills. The reader might care to spend a few minutes devising an analogous condition for Patel's treatment package.)

Clearly the results reported by Patel represent an important advance in behavioural control of hypertension, offering the first convincing demonstration that this form of treatment has clinical relevance. Within the context of the present discussion, two questions remain. What is it about the programme that produces such outstanding results, and which patients are likely to derive most benefit from this form of treatment?

The most striking difference between the early behavioural techniques and Patel's programme is the extent to which she involves the patients in their own treatment. For example, we are not normally invited to attend meetings with other patients in order to have our illness explained to us, and to discuss freely our queries and problems with the medical staff. Even less are we likely to be given access to our records. Furthermore, treatment does not end the minute the patient leaves the surgery. Rather, he is positively encouraged to incorporate what has been learned into his everyday life. Finally, and crucially, what he learns is a method whereby he, rather than the doctor, assumes responsibility for his health. Contrast this approach with the early applications of biofeedback, where the patient was attached to a piece of apparatus and 'left to get on with it'.

Without doubt, patient involvement is a factor which affects the outcome of this form of therapy. We have already seen that merely requiring patients to monitor their own blood pressure regularly has a significant effect on the efficacy of both meditation and biofeedback. Furthermore, Sherman and Gaardner (1977) have reported that a review of all the published studies involving biofeedback and meditation revealed a positive correlation between decreased blood pressure and degree of involvement. Why this should be so has still to be fully explained, but there are grounds for believing that involving the patient increases his motivation to comply with the treatment.

It is not difficult to see why poor compliance might be a problem with this form of therapy. For all the evidence shows that in order to remain effective, the 'relaxation response' must become a permanent feature of the patient's way of life. Yet any doctor knows how difficult it can be to persuade a patient to persevere with a long-term treatment regime, even when it is simple, and failure to do so produces overt symptoms. The task is infinitely greater when, as in this case, treatment is time consuming, and the condition frequently asymptomatic.

The extent to which motivation is central to Patel's programme is further illustrated by her use of biofeedback. The fact that she employed EMG and GSR, rather than direct feedback, suggests that they were regarded as an aid to deep relaxation, as much as therapeutic measures in their own right. This assumption received some support when Hafner (1982) demonstrated that the overall efficacy of the programme was not affected by omitting feedback, although the final outcome did take longer to achieve. However, this is not to devalue the contribution made by feedback. Many people find it virtually impossible to relax, and without the early success that feedback helps to make possible, they might well lose heart, and abandon the programme altogether. Thus not only does feedback help the patient learn to relax, but by doing so it acts as a further source of motivation to persevere with the treatment.

Concluding remarks

In a discussion of her own work, Patel proposed that relaxation-based behavioural methods might be offered as a first-line treatment to patients with mild hypertension. The weight of evidence justifies the conclusion, for her treatment has proved effective in enabling a significant minority of patients to abandon, or greatly reduce, hypertensive medication. At the same time, no one should be deceived into believing that this form of therapy is as wide ranging or powerful as conventional pharmacological treatment. We have already seen that hypertension due to vascular change is unlikely to respond to behavioural techniques, although sufferers might be offered a degree of protection from the stress-induced surge in pressure to which they are especially vulnerable.

Headache

Methodological problems

It might appear odd to begin a review of the behavioural control of headache with a discussion of methodological issues. However, as the preceding section highlighted, there are major methodological difficulties in investigating behavioural techniques in a manner which allows unequivocal statements to be made about their mode of action and efficacy. While such difficulties occur whatever the nature of the illness, they are especially hard to overcome in the case of headache, or indeed any pain state. For by its very nature, pain is a subjective experience which cannot be measured directly, but has to be inferred from the patient's verbal reports and general demeanour. Researchers and clinicians are, therefore, forced to rely upon indirect measures in order to obtain their data. These can range from a simple five-point rating scale, to complex questionnaires which seek to measure pain along a variety of dimensions. Other measures make no attempt to quantify subjective sensations, but rely upon observable behaviour, such as the amount of analgesia required over a given period of time.

Unfortunately, no single index of pain has gained universal acceptance, thus making comparisons between different studies well nigh impossible. For example, how are we to judge whether a treatment which reduces the mean daily pain rating from 4.40 to 1.84 is more effective than one which produces a reduction in medication of 56%; and to judge further whether both are better than a third treatment which reduces the frequency of occurrence of headaches from nine per week to two? Moreover, problems of measurement are not confined to comparisons between studies. For it is well established that pain has both affective and somatic properties (Melzack and Wall, 1979), and a clinician might easily be misled into believing that a therapy had dramatically reduced somatic pain, when in fact the patient had experienced relief from depression. The reader is urged to bear these problems in mind when attempting to make sense of the many contradictory findings that are reviewed in the next two sections.

Chronic headache

Because the condition is usually benign, and self-medication is freely available, it is difficult to estimate the incidence of chronic headache. However, as is pointed out in Macleod (1981), headache is the commonest, as well as one of the most ambiguous and difficult, problems in clinical medicine. Although headache is symptomatic of many diseases, the vast majority of chronic cases are diagnosed as either tension headache or migraine. Because they are so common, and are the two types of headache most frequently treated by behavioural techniques, the present discussion is confined to these two conditions.

Tension headache

Frequently the patient presenting with tension headache describes his symptoms as a tight band that circles the head, or a stretching of the skin, rather than as a definite pain. The Ad-hoc Committee on the Classification of Headache (1962) describes tension headache as being '... associated with sustained contraction of the skeletal muscles in the absence of permanent structural change, usually as part of the individual's reaction to life stress'. Faced with this description, it is hardly surprising that tension headache has become a prime target for behavioural techniques. For, while biofeedback offers a ready-made solution to the problem of specific muscle contraction, a programme of deep relaxation might allow the sufferer to reduce the underlying stress.

EMG feedback and tension headache

The principles governing the application of EMG feedback have already been outlined on page 118. Bearing in mind that this method allows the individual to learn to relax specific muscles, it is hardly surprising that it has been widely used to treat tension headache. However, before assessing clinical efficacy, we need to question the assumption that tension headache is caused by sustained muscular contraction. The search for verification has centred on two hypotheses:

1. during headache-free periods, sufferers will have higher levels of tension in the head muscles than will controls; and/or

2. sufferers will show increased activity in these muscles at the onset of a headache.

The first hypothesis was confirmed by Budzynski *et al.* (1973) who described how sufferers exhibited resting levels of frontalis activity which were twice those of controls. These findings were confirmed by van Boxtel and van der Ven (1978), who also reported that the effect was specific to the frontales, and did not represent a raised level of general muscular activity. The second hypothesis also received support when Haynes *et al.* (1975) reported that EMG levels rose during headache, confirming earlier findings by Sainsbury and Gibson (1954), who showed that frontalis activity increased relative to that in the arm. Although these four outcomes justify using EMG feedback to treat tension headache, there is at least one published study which urges caution. Bakal and Kaganov (1977) compared frontalis activity of controls with that of sufferers from either migraine or tension headache. Not only were levels highest in the migraine group, but there were no differences between control subjects and those with tension headache, even when at the time of measurement the latter were actually suffering from headache. Bearing in mind the methodological problems that beset this area of research, we should not be too surprised when such inconsistencies occur. On the other hand, there are no obvious methodological differences to account for the discrepancy between these findings and those described earlier.

Clinical outcome

One of the earliest successful applications of frontalis EMG feedback in the treatment of tension headache was demonstrated by Budzynski and his associates in the study discussed in the previous section. They reported how 16 treatment sessions, spread over a period of 8 weeks, produced a clinically significant decrease in headaches, with a concomitant decrease in frontalis activity. At the same time the use of analgesics and tranquillisers was greatly reduced, and there was a lessening of related symptoms such as anxiety, depression and insomnia. Similarly, Kondo and Canter (1977) found that frequency of headaches was reduced in 10 patients receiving EMG feedback, but not in controls who received false feedback. Unlike the early studies of biofeedback and hypertension, these findings were not to fail the test of replication. Several studies confirmed the value of EMG feedback, and subsequent research quickly turned from clinical evaluation to an examination of underlying mechanisms.

Not surprisingly, one of the first issues to attract attention concerned the extent to which reduction in headaches was due to specific EMG training, rather than to a more general relaxation effect. An early attempt to answer this question was reported by Haynes et al. (1975) in a study which has already been cited. They compared the effects of EMG feedback, relaxation training and an untreated control group. The results showed that although both treated groups did better than controls, when compared with each other there was no difference in outcome; frequency of headache being reduced by about 80% in each case. It is worth observing that such a large decrease would have masked any differences in efficacy that might exist between the two forms of treatment, and a study of very severe cases might well have produced a different outcome. This is, of course, mere speculation, and on balance the early studies suggested that in terms of final outcome, there was little to choose between EMG feedback and deep relaxation procedures. However, other findings indicated that the picture might not be so simple. For example, the original study of Budzynski *et al.* reported correlations between reduction in headache and decrease in frontalis activity to be 0.90; other workers have reported values as low as 0.42. (Indeed, there is at least one reported case of a decrease in headache being accompanied by increased EMG activity.)

This lack of consistency is in accord with the argument advanced by Dalessio (1972) that tension headache is, in fact, underlaid by more than one factor. Thus, although pain can arise from increased muscle contraction alone, it is more likely to occur, and with greater intensity, if the increase is accompanied by vasoconstriction. Moreover, as we shall see in the following section, peripheral vasoconstriction decreases during deep relaxation. The recognition that vascular factors are involved in tension headache is especially relevant to the present discussion on two counts. First, it explains the failure to find a consistent relationship between frontalis EMG activity and headache intensity; and second, it implies that EMG feedback and deep relaxation training might well have independent therapeutic roles. More precisely, relaxation will be especially effective in dealing with headaches in which there is an element of vasoconstriction, while feedback will enable the sufferer to overcome those in which the pain results from specific muscular contraction. One study has attempted to examine this hypothesis in detail.

Blanchard *et al.* (1982) proposed that if EMG feedback and deep relaxation operate differently, then patients who derived no benefit from one form of treatment might yet do so from the other. Fourteen sufferers from chronic tension headaches entered the study, beginning with a 4-week baseline period, followed by an 8-week programme of deep relaxation training, comprising ten 35-minute sessions. The technique was similar to those outlined earlier, emphasising the role of muscular relaxation, and control of breathing. At the end of the relaxation phase, the 14 patients entered a 12-session programme of frontalis EMG feedback, spread over a period of 6–12 weeks.

Throughout the programme subjects kept a 'headache diary', which allowed changes in symptoms to be measured using a variety of scales.

In summary, the results showed that by the end of the relaxation phase, 6 patients had reduced symptoms by more than 25% (mean 50.4%), 4 showed minimal or no change, while the remaining 4 showed increases in symptoms in excess of 25% (mean 51%). Following the subsequent EMG feedback, 5 patients had improved by more than 40% (mean 70.2%), *relative to their condition at the end of the relaxation phase*. Faced with this last finding, it is easy to believe that EMG feedback had indeed produced a degree of improvement which was not attainable by relaxation alone. However, an inspection of the individual data shows that 4 of these 5 patients had also improved significantly by the end of the relaxation phase (mean 49.3%). Thus, although further improvement might have been due to a unique effect of EMG feedback, it could equally represent a continuing effect of relaxation. This ambiguity could have been resolved had the study included a control group which carried on with relaxation when the experimental group switched to feedback training. Unfortunately this control was omitted, though it is interesting to observe that the four patients who gained no benefit from relaxation failed to benefit from EMG feedback either (mean 1%). This is a tantalising piece of research, for the omission of a control group prevents us from reaching some important conclusions about the specific effects of EMG feedback. As it is, the study demonstrated that:

(a) relaxation training alone can produce a significant reduction in tension headache, although not all sufferers benefit;

(b) certain individuals who fail to benefit from relaxation training are unlikely to benefit from EMG feedback;

(c) patients who benefit from relaxation training show further improvement following EMG feedback.

The reason for this additional improvement cannot be clearly specified, although it remains a possibility that these two forms of treatment differ in their modes of action.

There is one other aspect of this study which makes it worthy of detailed coverage. A further analysis was designed to investigate the characteristics of those patients who failed to derive benefit from treatment. It emerged that compared with those who obtained significant relief, 'failures' were more depressed, and showed a tendency to be more hysterical. This is an important finding to which we shall return later.

Long-term effects

In view of what was said earlier, it is not surprising to learn that therapeutic gains are maintained only if the patient continues to practise what was learned in the training sessions. Indeed, a 12-month follow-up study reported by Reinking and Hutchings (1981) suggests that long-term outcome depends more upon continued practice than on the initial method of learning. One of the largest follow-up studies (Diamond *et al.*, 1979) involved a postal survey of 556 patients who had undergone biofeedback training for either tension headache or migraine during the preceding 5 years. The results (based upon 407 replies) showed that 3 to 5 years after treatment, 62.6% of patients claimed that the treatment was effective, with 20.6% reporting permanent relief. It is interesting that these authors also report that depression and drug dependency are contraindications for this form of therapy.

Concluding remarks

It will have become apparent that there is still a great deal to be discovered about tension headache *per se*, as well as the role of EMG feedback and deep relaxation in its treatment. I have deliberately emphasised the fact that there are many questions still to be answered; largely to counteract some of the extravagant claims that are all too frequently made on behalf of these forms of therapy. On the other hand, it would be unfortunate if the reader were left with the impression that here is an interesting area of research that sometime in the future might have a clinical application.

There is already ample evidence to show that both EMG feedback and deep relaxation training have a major part to play in the treatment of tension headache, and in a significant number of cases offer a real alternative to conventional pharmacological methods. In common with all behavioural self-control techniques, motivation will be a significant factor in determining outcome, although the fact that headache answers non-compliance with unpleasant symptoms suggests that maintaining motivation might be less of a problem than it is in treating mild hypertension.

As the preceding section emphasised, the choice of treatment will depend upon the nature of the tension headache. Where stress and vasoconstriction predominate, some form of deep relaxation training is appropriate, while EMG feedback is more suitable for those cases in which severe muscular spasm is the underlying cause.

Migraine headache

Although in everyday usage the term migraine is synonymous with a particular type of headache, on closer examination it soon becomes apparent that we are dealing with a complex phenomenon, which can take a variety of forms. Quite apart from migrainous neuralgia (also known as cluster headache), Blau (1982) has proposed that it is possible to identify six variants, and even the simplest clinical classification distinguishes between classic and common migraine. Because common migraine can be regarded as a lesser version of classic migraine, only the latter will be discussed in detail.

Classic migraine

The term classic migraine refers to that condition in which the headache is preceded by a number of well-defined symptoms. This period, known as the prodromal stage (Greek *prodromos*, running before), can last up to 12 hours, and is often characterised by changes in mood, a craving for certain foods, and retention of fluid. Towards the end of the prodromal stage, aura may develop in the form of flashes of light, and restriction of the visual field. (It should be noted that aura does not invariably occur in migraine, and Blau has suggested that it is absent in up to 80% of cases.) Aura rarely lasts for more than 1 hour, before giving way to the headache stage.

Initially, the headache may be mild and localised to a small spot, before developing into a throbbing pain which is made worse by movement and is often confined to one side of the head. At the same time many sufferers develop nausea, and a significant number prefer to avoid bright lights. This stage is of variable duration, but it is often terminated by sleep, although for 2 or 3 days thereafter the sufferer may continue to feel lethargic and mildly depressed.

The cause of migraine

To ascribe causal properties to any agent implies that the underlying mechanisms are fully understood. In the case of migraine this is not so, and it is safer, therefore, to talk of *precipitating* factors. These have been shown to be wide ranging and include: dietary factors (especially foods such as chocolate, cheese, red wines and citrus fruits); low levels of blood sugar; hormonal changes (especially those associated with the menstrual cycle and the contraceptive pill); allergy; changes in patterns of sleep; loud noise and bright lights; a wide range of psychological factors, including both increased and decreased levels of stress. It needs to be emphasised that not all sufferers respond to the same precipitating factors, nor will a particular factor necessarily trigger an attack in the same individual on every occasion.

Underlying mechanism

Given that it takes more than one form, and is precipitated by so many factors, it is hardly surprising that no single theory has satisfactorily explained every aspect of migraine, although the vascular theory remains dominant. However, even this theory exists in a number of forms, and what follows is no more than a simplified outline, the purpose of which is to enable the reader to appreciate the rationale for treating migraine by behavioural means.

The theory argues that a precipitating factor leads to vasoconstriction within the carotid or vertebrobasilar vascular tree. It is believed that vasoconstriction involves a number of biochemical changes, of which an increase in the level of serotonin is especially important. The initial vasoconstriction produces symptoms of ischaemia within the brain cells, before giving way to vasodilatation within the intra- and extracranial arteries. Vasodilatation corresponds to the headache stage, which is believed to arise from the stretching of nerve endings within the walls of the arteries. It must be added that biochemical changes that accompany migraine are not restricted to those involving serotonin, but also include fluctuations in the levels of histamine, prostaglandins, bradykinin, adrenaline and noradrenaline (Melzak and Wall, 1979).

Despite being an oversimplification, the above outline

suggests that the treatment of migraine can be approached from a number of directions. These will focus on precipitating factors, vascular changes, and the provision of symptomatic pain relief. Not surprisingly, conventional treatment relies heavily on pharmacological control, which includes preventing vasoconstriction by administering a serotonin antagonist such as methysergide, or much more commonly by prescribing ergotamine to combat vasodilatation. The precipitating factors are obviously best dealt with by avoiding them, though the benzodiazepines are occasionally used to reduce the effects of stress.

Behavioural control of migraine

As with pharmacological methods, so the behavioural techniques used to control migraine have varied, depending upon which component is being treated. In those cases where stress and anxiety are found to be major precipitating factors various programmes of deep relaxation have been employed with some success. However, as with tension headaches (but unlike hypertension), the majority of research has centred upon one form of biofeedback.

Temperature feedback

Whatever views we might hold about the efficacy of EMG feedback, few would dispute that there is a certain logic in its use to treat tension headache. However, it is much less obvious why temperature feedback should be used to control migraine, especially when the method involves learning to raise the temperature of the finger or hand. In fact this particular application was not based upon any theoretical premise, but arose out of a chance observation made by Sargent *et al.* (1972). They described how a subject spontaneously recovered from an attack of migraine while she was learning to control EEG patterns, reduce EMG activity in the forearm, and increase blood flow to the hands. At the same time, the temperature of the hand, *relative to the forehead*, rose by 10°F. This single observation was to produce a flood of clinical trials which appeared to show that feedback-assisted hand warming offered a powerful new method of treating migraine. Before turning to these studies, however, we need to examine the assumptions that were made about this peculiar phenomenon.

Sargent *et al.* proposed that the effect was due to a reduction in sympathetic outflow, rather than to a 'hydraulic maneuvering of blood in various portions of the body'. This is an appealing hypothesis, for as we have seen, one effect of increased SNS output is a raised level of catecholamines, as part of the more general fight or flight response. Furthermore, a finding reported by Henryk-Gutt and Rees (1973), that migraine sufferers have increased scores on the neuroticism scale of the Eysenck Personality Inventory, suggests that the condition is associated with a labile ANS. These observations led Yates (1980) to propose that migraine sufferers are particularly prone to increased SNS output when faced with stress. As a consequence there is an increase in serotonin secretion, which in turn leads to vasoconstriction, thus triggering the cycle outlined earlier. Although this account accords with much of the data, two comments are necessary. First, although increased stress frequently does precipitate an attack of migraine in certain individuals, we have already seen that an attack can also follow a *reduction* in stress. In the latter case the role of serotonin is far from clear. Second, a correlation between neuroticism and migraine activity has not been unequivocally demonstrated, and at least one survey failed to find any such relationship.

Clinical outcome

Following the single case study referred to earlier, Sargent *et al.* produced a number of reports suggesting that temperature feedback training was effective in treating migraine, with success rates as high as 74% being reported. Unfortunately these studies were open to the almost routine criticism of poor design, so that Yates (1980) has described them as being of only historical interest. Despite such criticisms, most of the early trials achieved similar success rates, so that more complex investigations began to emerge. These sought not only to measure clinical outcome in a more rigorous fashion, but also to identify the key factors underlying this form of treatment.

One of the more interesting of these studies was reported by Johnson and Turin (1975). They used continuous visual feedback in order to train a subject first to cool her fingers, then to warm them. Each phase lasted for 6 weeks, during which time the subject was encouraged to expect success. The results showed that compared with baseline, cooling produced an increase in migraine activity, whereas warming had the opposite effect. A subsequent study which employed seven subjects produced a similar outcome. In so far as increased finger temperature reflects decreased SNS output, these findings support the hypothesis that a reduction in SNS activity is commensurate with a reduction in migraine. However, subsequent studies were to reveal that this is only a small part of the story. For example, Mullinix *et al.* (1978) found that reductions in headache occurred irrespective of whether the patient was given true or false feedback. Even more confusing was the finding reported by Kewman and Roberts (1980), that raising and lowering the temperature of the hand were equally effective forms of treatment, but no more so than simply requiring patients to keep records of migraine activity.

What makes this study novel is the fact that neither the subjects nor their therapists were aware to which of the two experimental conditions they had been assigned. In the words of the authors:

Subjects were not told whether they were being trained to increase or decrease finger temperature. Rather they were simply told to respond to a tone, a meter, or both, which registered relative changes in finger temperature with no information regarding whether they were being trained to increase or decrease temperature.

The whole programme lasted 21 weeks, consisting of a 6-week baseline phase, a 9-week treatment phase (comprising ten 1-hour training sessions) and a 6-week follow-up phase. Throughout the 21-week period, all subjects kept diaries in which they recorded detailed information about their attacks of migraine. The results showed that by the end of the follow-up phase, all three groups had undergone significant reductions in severity of attacks, number of symptoms, and amount of medication. There were similar, though non-significant, trends in both frequency and duration of attacks for all three groups. Surprisingly, however, there were no significant differences between the three groups on any of the five measures. In other words, although finger warming produced reductions in migraine activity that were statistically and clinically significant, identical effects were achieved simply by requiring patients to keep detailed records of their attacks.

These studies are especially interesting in that they demonstrate the multiplicity of factors that underlie the successful treatment of migraine by behavioural methods. Thus, Kewman and Roberts (1980) concluded that the outcome of their study could only be explained in terms of non-specific factors, such as increased doctor–patient rapport. On the other hand, it is difficult to interpret the positive effects reported by Johnson and Turin in this way. For, by leading subjects to believe that cooling and warming the hand would relieve symptoms, they provided an effective control for non-specific factors. However, even if we accept that in this case reduction in symptoms was directly linked to hand warming, it does not follow that a similar outcome could not have been achieved by other means. Indeed, it appears that any method which reduces SNS output will help at least a proportion of migraine sufferers. For example, Hay and Madders (1971) reported a 70% improvement rate following a programme of relaxation training. Moreover, Blanchard *et al.* (1978) found no difference in outcome in a comparison of finger temperature feedback and systematic relaxation training. Immediately following cessation of treatment, those subjects trained in relaxation showed the greater improvement, although 1 year later this difference was no longer present; both groups continuing to exhibit a significant reduction in symptoms (Silver *et al.*, 1979). Given the complex nature of migraine, it is perhaps surprising to find behavioural treatments producing such encouraging long-term effects. Yet the outcome reported by Silver *et al.* does not appear to be exceptional. Indeed, a comprehensive review of the literature by Ford (1982) indicates that the long-term success rate is greater for vascular headache (70%) than it is for tension headache (50%).

Concluding remarks

The studies reviewed in this section have reported some outcomes that are contradictory, and many that are perplexing. Yet amidst this confusion one finding is clear: a significant number of migraine sufferers have been shown to obtain considerable relief following either temperature feedback or relaxation training. Moreover, the limited number of follow-up studies that have been published indicate that the effect is relatively long lasting. What is not clear is the precise nature of the mechanisms by which these clinically significant effects were achieved.

Because migraine exists in so many forms, and is precipitated by such a wide range of factors, plus the fact that pain has emotional as well as sensory qualities, it should come as no surprise to find that biofeedback and relaxation training operate at more than one level. Already the work of Kewman and Roberts (1980) has pointed to the importance of non-specific factors in treating migraine. Their conclusions resemble those reached by Patel, which emphasised the crucial role of motivation and self-determination in the relaxation-based behavioural methods. So far, neither migraine nor tension headache has been treated in the comprehensive manner that Patel brought to bear on hypertension. This is a pity, for, unlike essential hypertension, there is no evidence that these two conditions produce permanent structural changes, and consequently we could hope for higher success rates. Just as we need to know more about the way in which non-specific effects might be turned to clinical advantage, so more research is needed into the specific effects of reducing SNS activity.

Before moving on to a general summary, there is one other application of biofeedback which must be mentioned. A number of attempts have been made to train migraine sufferers to control directly constriction of cranial blood vessels. Unfortunately discussion of these studies is beyond the scope of this chapter, and the interested reader should consult Yates (1980).

Summary

This discussion has been limited to essential hypertension and headache to enable the mechanisms underlying biofeedback and meditation to be examined in some detail. What, then, have we learned about these two treatments?

We began by arguing that there are good grounds for believing that many non-infectious diseases are intimately associated with the stresses of modern-day living. It was further argued that an important contributor to this association is an inappropriately high level of SNS output. Given these assumptions, it follows that any method which enables autonomic activity to be controlled should be of value in treating stress-related illnesses. The studies reviewed here, though often ambiguous, show that this is so, both biofeedback and deep relaxation training producing clinically significant improvements. With hypertension these tend to be modest and difficult to maintain, whereas tension headache and migraine respond much more favourably. However, whatever the magnitude of these successful outcomes, it became increasingly obvious that they were the result of some extremely complex mechanisms.

The first point to emerge is that when applied to stress-linked diseases, biofeedback operates in a manner which owes more to general relaxation than to the control of a specific autonomic response. Moreover, although the decrease in SNS activity that accompanies deep relaxation training is an important component of this form of therapy, it is now widely accepted that cognitive factors are equally important. Thus, it became necessary to import into the discussion terms such as motivation, doctor–patient rapport, and self-perception in order to make sense of seemingly contradictory data. (It is necessary to pause here and point out that not every successful application of biofeedback is underlaid by a general relaxation effect. We have already seen that headache due to muscle contraction would be expected to show a specific response to EMG feedback. Similarly, EMG feedback is used to help retrain individual muscle movements following injury to the neuromuscular system. Clearly, in this case feedback is filling a role which could not be undertaken by relaxation training.)

Returning to the stress-linked illnesses, I have allowed myself the luxury of an anecdotal case study in order to illustrate the importance of cognitive factors. Recently I was asked to treat a man in his early thirties who for the last 2 years had suffered from overwhelming attacks of anxiety. While there was no apparent reason for these atacks, they had reached a level where there was a danger that he would become a chronic agoraphobic. A treatment programme very similar to that devised by Patel was constructed, comprising: a 4-week programme of GSR-assisted relaxation training, using the technique devised by Benson *et al.* (see page 111); regular practice at home throughout the 4 weeks (including GSR feedback); the keeping of daily diaries in which the patient rated his level of anxiety, and noted any occasions when he was especially anxious. From the outset he was encouraged to try to carry over into his daily life what he learned at the clinic, especially when faced with stress.

By the end of the fourth week there was a marked reduction in the anxiety ratings, and the patient claimed to be coping much better, describing his improvement as follows:

Relaxation has taught me to control my anxiety ... I'm not frightened to go out now in case I have an attack ... I would know how to relax ... I understand what's happening now ... it's odd really, if I get an attack I control my breathing, and I can almost hear that machine stop clicking.

This case was not presented in order to demonstrate that chronic anxiety responds to relaxation-based behavioural treatment (although there is evidence to show that it does). It was introduced as a simple example of the complex interaction of physiological and cognitive factors that are involved in the behavioural control of stress-related illnesses.

As the patient's own words make clear, his perceptions of himself and his environment are changing—he became able to control his anxiety and to understand what was happening. This has led him to face the outside world, and to learn that he is not going to die in the middle of a crowded pavement. Moreover, with this new-found confidence he claims to be coping better with pressures at home and at work. Clearly there is much more happening here than can be attributed to conditioning of an autonomic response, or damping down the ANS. Yet, at the same time, this patient insists that without the initial biofeedback-assisted relaxation training, he would never have been able to go on and bring about the other changes.

Obtaining treatment

A medical practitioner wishing to refer patients for this form of treatment is likely to face a number of difficulties. First, there is no professional register of individuals who have undertaken specific training in biofeedback and/or meditation. The nearest approximation to such a register is probably the list of members eligible for entry to the Clinical Division of the British Psychological Society. Despite the recent trend for clinical psychologists to find employment in health centres, it still remains the case that the majority are employed in psychiatric hospitals, neurological units or hospitals for the subnormal. Nevertheless, a practitioner requiring guidance in the use of these forms of therapy should consider seeking the advice of a local clinical psychologist. He must recognise, however, that not all clinical psychologists utilise biofeedback or meditation in their daily practice.

When we turn to private practitioners, the position becomes extremely complicated. At present anyone can offer his services as a psychologist, with no restrictions on advertising. This is an unfortunate state of affairs which has attracted its share of charlatans. It would be wise, therefore, to ask anyone claiming to be a psychologist if he is eligible for membership of the British Psychological Society.

The second major difficulty is less concerned with the availability of outside practitioners than it is with the therapeutic value of such referrals. Patel argues (and her achievements suggest she is correct) that if the treatment is to be fully effective it needs to be carried out by the patient's own doctor as part of an integrated programme. In particular, motivation is much less likely to be maintained if the patient is 'packed off to someone down the road' to undergo biofeedback-assisted relaxation training. Thus the doctor most likely to achieve success with this form of treatment is the one who either administers it himself or entrusts it to someone who is an active and involved member of his practice.

Finally a word about equipment. It is possible to spend enormous sums of money on biofeedback monitoring equipment. Although precisely tuned equipment may be necessary in the research laboratory, its use in clinical practice is rarely justified. Indeed, some laboratory instruments which measure changes in single muscle fibres would be inappropriate for measuring gross changes in the musculature of, say, the head and neck. Similar remarks apply to GSR monitors, where it should not be necessary to spend more than £60–£70 to obtain a perfectly adequate machine.

Contraindications and side-effects

It was argued earlier in this chapter that the behavioural techniques are of very limited value in conditions such as secondary hypertension, where permanent structural changes have occurred. However, the preceding discussion suggests another category of patient who will fail to benefit from this form of therapy. In this case the reason lies not so much in the patient's vascular system as in his mental outlook. He is the individual who regards all illness as something to be dealt with by the medical profession and will look askance at the suggestion that he, rather than the doctor, should control his symptoms. In principle it ought to be possible to detect such patients before offering them this form of therapy. Currently, this research is in its infancy, though we have already seen that depressed or hysterical individuals achieve relatively poor outcomes. Indeed, there are grounds for arguing that biofeedback is contraindicated where the condition is a product of deep psychological conflicts. The complicated electronic gadgetry employed in biofeedback can all too easily lead this type of patient to externalise his symptoms, rather than seeking to resolve the underlying problems.

There are two other groups of patients with whom these techniques should be used with care: epileptics, and those with a history of psychotic illness. Donaldson and Fenwick (1982) described how grand mal seizures are an acknowledged side-effect in epileptic meditators. They also point out that some teachers of meditation actually regard the seizures as a beneficial discharge of stress, and an indication for further meditation! Clearly there is a need for epileptics to approach meditation with extreme caution (and to be particularly wary of cranks who teach that grand mal is a favourable sign).

Similar problems have been encountered by individuals with a history of schizophrenia. Walsh and Roche (1979) have described how three such individuals developed acute psychotic symptoms following prolonged periods of meditation. It is worth pointing out that the authors concluded that:

These cases suggest that the combination of intensive meditation, fasting, sleep deprivation, a history of schizophrenia, and the discontinuation of maintenance doses of phenothiazines can be hazardous.

Clearly such a regime is quite unlike the programmes that have been described in this chapter. However, feelings of unreality and depersonalisation can accompany most forms of deep relaxation. As these feelings can prove disturbing, prudence dictates that patients with a history of psychotic illness should not be encouraged to undertake meditation, except under supervision.

Finally, while recognising the existence of these side-effects, they need to be kept in perspective. Certainly they pale into insignificance when compared with those associated with pharmacological treatments. Moreover, simply to compare the two forms of treatment in this way is to overlook the principal advantage of the behavioural techniques. For, when applied successfully, their effects extend beyond the condition being treated, so that the patient will have taken the first steps in learning to combat a whole range of stress-linked illnesses.

References

Ad-hoc Committee on the Classification of Headache (1962). Classification of headache. *Journal of American Medical Association*; **179**:717–18.

Bakal D. A., Kaganov J. A. (1977). Muscle contraction and migraine headache: psychophysiologic comparison. *Headache*; **17**:208–14.

Basmajian J. V., ed. (1983). *Biofeedback Principles and Practice for Clinicians*. Baltimore/London: Williams and Wilkins.

Benson H., Kotch J. B., Crassweller K. D., Greenwood M. M. (1977). Historical and clinical considerations of the relaxation response. *American Scientist*; **65**:441–5.

Blackwell B., Hanenson I., Bloomfield S. *et al.* (1976). Transcendental meditation in hypertension: individual response patterns. *Lancet*; **1**:223–6.

Blanchard E.B. (1979). Biofeedback and the modification of cardiovascular dysfunctions. In *Clinical Applications of Biofeedback: Appraisal and Status* (Gatchel, R. J., Price, K. P., eds.) pp. 28–51. Oxford: Pergamon Press.

Blanchard E. B., Andrasik F., Neff D. F. *et al.* (1982). Sequential comparisons of relaxation training and biofeedback in the treatment of three kinds of chronic headache or, the machines may be necessary some of the time. *Behaviour Research Therapy*; **20**:469–81.

Blanchard E. B., Theobold D. E., Williamson D. A., Silver B. V., Brown D. A. (1978). Temperature feedback in the treatment of migraine headache. *Archives of General Psychiatry*; **35**:581–8.

Blau J. N. (1982). *Migraine*. London: Update Publications.

van Boxtel A., van der Ven J. R. (1978). Differential EMG activity in subjects with muscle contraction headaches related to mental effort. *Headache*; **17**:233–7.

Budzynski T. H., Stoyva J. M., Adler C. S., Mullaney D. J. (1973). EMG biofeedback and tension headache: a controlled outcome study. *Psychosomatic Medicine*; **35**:484–96.

Dalessio D. J. (1972). *Wolff's Headache and Other Head Pain*, 3rd edn. New York: Oxford University Press.

Diamond S. M. D., Medina J. M. D., Diamond-Falk J. B. A., De Veno T. B. S. (1979). The value of biofeedback in the treatment of chronic headache: a five-year retrospective study. *Headache*; **19**:90–96.

Donaldosn S., Fenwick P. B. C. (1982). Effects of meditation. *American Journal of Psychiatry*; **139**:1217.

Fenwick P. (1983). Can we still recommend meditation? *British Medical Journal*; **287**:1401.

Ford M. R. (1982). Biofeedback treatment for headache, Raynauds' disease, essential hypertension, and irritable bowel syndrome: a review of the long-term follow-up literature. *Biofeedback and Self-Regulation*; 7(4):521–36.

Hafner R. J. (1982). Psychological treatment of essential hypertension: a controlled comparison of meditation and meditation plus biofeedback. *Biofeedback and Self-Regulation*; 7, No. 3:305–16.

Hay K. M., Madders J. (1971). Migraine treated by relaxation therapy. *Journal of the Royal College of General Practitioners*; **21**:664–9.

Haynes S. N., Griffin P., Mooney D., Parise M. (1975). Electromyographic biofeedback and relaxation instructions in the treatment of muscle contraction headaches. *Behaviour Therapy*; **6**:672–8.

Henryk-Gutt R., Rees W. L. (1973). Psychological aspects of migraine. *Journal of Psychosomatic Research*; **17**:141–53.

Johnson W. G., Turin A. (1975). Biofeedback treatment of migraine headache: a systematic case study. *Behaviour Therapy*; **6**:394–7.

Kewman D., Roberts A. H. (1980). Skin temperature biofeedback and migraine headaches. A double-blind study. *Biofeedback and Self-Regulation*; **5**, No. 3:327–45.

Kondo C., Canter A. (1977). True and false electromyographic feedback: effect of tension headache. *Journal of Abnormal Psychology*; **86**:93–5.

Kristt D. A., Engel B. T. (1975). Learned control of blood pressure in patients with high blood pressure. *Circulation*; **51**:370–78.

Liddell H. S. (1934). The conditioned reflex. In *Comparative Psychology* (Moss F. A., ed.). Englewood Cliffs, N. J.: Prentice-Hall.

Macleod J., ed. (1981) *Davidson's Principles and Practice of Medicine*. Edinburgh: Churchill Livingstone.

Melzack R., Wall P. (1979). *The Challenge of Pain*. Harmondsworth: Penguin.

Miller N. E. (1972). Learning of visceral and glandular responses: postscript. In *Current Status of Physiological Psychology: Readings* (Singh D., Morgan C. T., eds.) pp. 245–50. Monterey: Brooks/Cole.

Miller N. E. (1978). Biofeedback and visceral learning. In *Annual Review of Psychology* (Rosenzweig M. R., Porter L. W., eds.). Palo Alto, Calif.: Annual Reviews.

Mullinix J. M., Norton B. J., Hack S., Fishman M. A. (1978). Skin temperature, biofeedback and migraine. *Headache*; **17**:242–4.

Patel C., North W. R. S. (1975). Randomised controlled trial of yoga and biofeedback in management of hypertension. *Lancet*; **2**:93–5.

Pollack A. A., Weber M. A., Case D. B., Laragh J. H. (1977). Limitations of transcendental meditation in the treatment of essential hypertension. *Lancet*; **1**:71–3.

Reinking R. H., Hutchings D. (1981). Follow-up to: 'Tension headaches: what form of therapy is most effective?' *Biofeedback and Self-Regulation*; **6**, No. 1:57–62.

Sainsbury P., Gibson J. G. (1954). Symptoms of anxiety and tension and the accompanying physiological changes in the muscular system. *Journal of Neurology, Neuro-Surgery and Psychiatry*; **17**:216–24.

Sargent J. D., Green E. E., Walters E. D. (1972). The use of autogenic feedback training in a pilot study of migraine and tension headache. *Headache*; **12**:120–25.

Seer P. (1979). Psychological control of essential hypertension: review of the literature and methodological critique. *Psychological Bulletin*; **86**, No.5:1015–43.

Shapiro D. H. (1982). Overview: clinical and physiological comparison of meditation with other self-control strategies. *American Journal of Psychiatry*; **139**,3:267–74.

Sherman R. A., Gaardner K. R. (1977). *Patient Involvement and Treatment Effectiveness in Behavioural Treatments of Hypertension*. Paper presented at the meeting of the Biofeedback Society of America, Orlando.

Silver B. V., Blanchard E. B., Williamson D. A., Theobold D. E., Brown D. A. (1979). Temperature biofeedback and relaxation training in the treatment of migraine headaches. *Biofeedback and Self-Regulation*; **4**:359–66.

Walsh R., Roche L. (1979). The precipitation of acute psychotic episodes by intensive meditation in individuals with a history of schizophrenia. *American Journal of Psychiatry*; **136**:1085–6.

Yates A. J. (1980). *Biofeedback and the Modification of Behaviour*. New York: Plenum Press.

Useful addresses

British Society of Medical and Dental Hypnosis
c/o Mrs N. Samuels (Secretary for Metropolitan Branch)
42 Links Road
Ashtead
Surrey KT21 2AJ.

British Psychological Society
48 Princess Road East
Leicester LE1 7DR.
(Section for Clinical Psychologists: for attention of Mrs Bull.)

Chapter 4

Homoeopathic medicine
H. Boyd

In recent years there has been a growing interest in so-called alternative therapies for the treatment of patients, and these therapies cover a wide range of techniques, each with its own distinctive method and its own particular field of action. Many doctors are still unaware that homoeopathy is available within the National Health Service and that the hospitals and some clinics are a part of that service, financed by government and free to patients. The remedies used are prescribable in hospital or in general practice in the same way as conventional drugs. While there is a widespread use of homoeopathy by the public and an increasing number of lay practitioners setting up in private practice, the official body for training doctors in the use of homoeopathy is the Faculty of Homoeopathy. The faculty is recognised by Act of Parliament, and teaches qualified physicians in postgraduate study, with a diploma of membership by examination (MFHom.).

What is homoeopathy and why is it not taught in the undergraduate curriculum or more widely accepted by the medical profession? Homoeopathy is a system of therapeutics based on the use of the similar principle, the word being derived from the Greek words for similar (or like) and suffering. Dr Samuel Hahnemann, the founder of homoeopathy, observed that there were three ways in which to treat disease.

1. To find the cause and remove it. (Hence his important contributions to hygiene and public health.)
2. To treat by using 'contraries' or opposites—allopathy: an analgesic for pain, a sedative for sleep, a purgative for constipation. The term allopathy is largely outdated because much of

modern medicine depends on attacking organisms, or correcting biochemical and physiological changes, rather than prescribing direct opposites, although these are still used.

3. To use homoeopathic or similar remedies capable of producing an artificial illness similar in its symptomatology to the illness presented by the patient, and in this way cause the patient to react by means of his own defence mechanism, and so bring about recovery.

Hahnemann maintained that the use of 'allopathy' was acceptable in some acute states, of short duration, but in chronic illness this method was suppressant and led to other more deep-seated problems.

In conventional medicine we seek to find a cause for disease and if possible remove it. Failing this we try to make a diagnosis based on physiological symptoms and signs, backed up by investigation and study of pathology. There may then be a specific form of treatment, or we may require to use symptomatic remedies to relieve symptoms. In most situations our attention is disease orientated, and often localised to specific parts or organs, but frequently the uniquely individual response of the patient to his illness, and the overall effect of this illness on the patient, are sadly neglected.

If we look carefully at patients, even in acute disease with the same presenting pathology, it is possible to detect some symptoms which are characteristic of a particular person in his reaction to his illness, as well as those relating to the pathology. The homoeopathic doctor will place much more emphasis on these individual reactions in selecting his remedy, although he still requires to make a pathological diagnosis. In conventional medicine drugs are prescribed because their chemical constituents in some way influence the body's cells and tissues, and in most instances their toxic effects must be balanced against their therapeutic effects. The homoeopathic materia medica is largely composed of naturally occurring substances, as opposed to synthetic ones, but the toxicological effects are used to present a 'drug picture' of that substance. By studying the individual toxicology of each remedy, both in its known gross reactions and by observing the effect of administering repeated small doses of the remedy to healthy volunteers (proving), it is possible to build up a symptom-complex characteristic of that remedy.

When the symptom-complex of the patient is compared with the symptom-complexes of many remedies, it is often possible to find a close resemblance between the patient's total symptom picture and that of a single remedy. This remedy will be the 'similar remedy' then used in homoeopathic treatment.

Although there is still much scepticism and opposition to the concept of the use of 'similars' (or homoeopathy), it is interesting to note that this method is also employed in conventional prescribing: amphetamine (a stimulant) for treating a hyperactive child; digitalis, which in its overdosage produces similar symptoms to those which we use it to treat; x-ray and radium, which both cause and cure cancer; vaccines, which are made from tissue products and used to raise the patient's resistance to infection with the same organism.

Is the concept of homoeopathic prescribing really so strange and impossible? Those who use homoeopathic remedies selected carefully for the individual patient frequently find that these remedies will clear up acute common illnesses quickly and safely without the need for conventional drugs. In conditions requiring surgery, homoeopathic physicians use remedies before and after operations, but the indications for surgery are the same. In certain deficiency states conventional replacement therapy is necessary and drugs such as thyroxine, insulin, vitamin B12, iron or steroids should be prescribed in normal dosage.

In some severe infections, such as meningitis, tuberculosis, septicaemia or venereal disease, most homoeopathic doctors use conventional antibiotics. It should be emphasised that homoeopathy does not consist of giving conventional drugs in ridiculously small doses. The use of highly diluted solutions or potencies is confined to the homoeopathic remedies prescribed on the similar principle.

In chronic disease homoeopathy can sometimes achieve remarkable improvement, or alleviation when various forms of conventional therapy have failed to help. In certain cases both types of therapy may be used to complement each other. A patient with severe rheumatoid arthritis may still require an analgesic or non-steroidal anti-rheumatic drug as well as his homoeopathic remedies, or an asthmatic patient may require inhalers. But with successful homoeopathic prescribing it may be possible to reduce other medication and to stop administration of drugs which cause unpleasant side-effects.

The developement of homoeopathy and the materia medica

The use of similar prescribing has been known for many hundreds of years, but the careful clinical application of homoeopathy first evolved by the observations and clinical trials conducted by Samuel Hahnemann in Germany around 1810 (Cook, 1981). It is interesting to note that the use of homoeopathy was not based on vague theories but on sound clinical observation and experiment. Hahnemann's studies began on cinchona bark (from which quinine is derived) and on mercury, both of which were used in fairly toxic doses for treatment in his day. He observed that the symptoms of 'marsh fever', for which cinchona was used, could be produced in himself and his colleagues by taking small amounts of an infusion of the bark. In other words, what this remedy could cause it could also cure. He experimented further with other plants, salts and metals, administering small quantities repetitively to healthy subjects and recording the toxic and side-effects of each substance. These tests were known as 'provings'. He then studied his patients and found that in certain illnesses a symptom picture was produced which closely resembled a drug picture from his provings and known toxicology. This remedy was then prescribed for that patient, often with remarkable results.

Much of the prescribing at this date was for acute epidemic disease, and his method proved vastly superior to the elaborate mixtures of numerous plants used by his colleagues. He wrote his *Organon of the Healing Art* in 1810, of which recent translations make interesting reading (Hahnemann, 1982). His understanding of disease and observations on hygiene and public health were remarkable for his time.

These provings and studies of remedies continued and a large materia medica was built up in Europe and then in America and in the United Kingdom. The practice of homoeopathy spread to many parts of the world and was brought to England by Dr Harvey Quin, who founded the Homoeopathic Hospital in London in 1850. Men like Hering, Dunham and Kent developed homoeopathy in the United States, and evolved their own methods of prescribing. Homoeopathy is widely used in the countries of Europe, in the Indian subcontinent and in South America.

The present-day materia medica of the homoeopathic doctor still contains all the original 'drug pictures' obtained from provings and toxicology, but has been enlarged with further remedies and also the addition of symptoms which were observed to disappear on giving a particular remedy to a number of patients. The remedies are prepared from plants, salts, minerals, venom of snakes and spiders, and many toxic substances. In recent years preparations from tissues or discharges (nosodes) have been added, and now remedies made from allergens such as house dust, cat and dog hair, grass pollens and moulds. These are used rather like vaccines to reduce the sensitivity of the allergic patient to particular substances. The original Latin names are retained because they are recognised internationally in any language and also because provings were often carried out on whole plants or minerals with other trace elements and not on purified extracts. Names like *Natrum muriaticum* (sodium chloride from rock salt), or *Silica* (silica and other trace minerals) or *Lachesis* (from the venom of the bushmaster snake) are well known in homoeopathy.

Some plant extracts are used in mother tinctures, like *Calendula* or *Crataegus*, but the vast majority are prepared by a special technique, called potentisation, in which quite infinitesimal doses are used. This process and the use of these seemingly impossible small quantities are the biggest stumbling blocks to acceptance of homoeopathy in medical and scientific circles. So here we have the second reason why homoeopathy is not more widely used and taught. How can a highly diluted solution have anything other than a placebo effect?

Potencies and infinitesimal dose

It is important to understand that these preparations are not simply straight dilutions, nor is their use the basis of the homoeopathic (similar) principle. The selection of the remedy on the matching of the patient's symptom picture with the remedy picture is paramount. However, the use of 'potencies' is part of everyday homoeopathic pharmacy. The term potency is used because the method of preparation seems to enhance the action of the remedy, giving it more 'power'. Plants are collected in the growing state from all parts of the world, under certain conditions of cultivation or in the wild. These are then crushed and an alcoholic extract obtained by soaking and filtering. The mother tincture is then diluted with 40% alcohol in strict proportions of 1 drop of tincture to either 10 or 100 drops of diluent. This vial is then shaken or succussed by hand or machine. One drop of this diluent is then transferred to the next vial of diluent containing 9 or 99 drops, and succussed. Each stage is designated 1 × (D, decimal) or 1C (centesimal). Two stages of 1 in 10 dilution with succussion would be 2 ×; three stages of 1 in 100 dilution with succussion would be 3C potency. This process is repeated up to 6 × or 12 × in the decimal range, or with centesimal dilutions to 30C or 200C or even higher (1M being 1000C).

In the case of insoluble substances, these are ground up with mortar and pestle using lactose as a diluent. The proportions are again 1 in 10. After thorough grinding (trituration) for several hours to break up and distribute the agent, a further 1 in 10 dilution is made with lactose, and grinding repeated. After three stages (3 × potency) this mixture can be suspended in alcohol and water and potentised as described for tinctures.

Attempts are now being made to standardise mother tinctures, as these do vary in different countries. Dr G. Jolliffe of the Pharmacy Department, University of London, has made a detailed study of the plants, first to identify the various species and then, by means of thin-layer chromatography, to isolate the various constituents. The manufacturing pharmacists in the UK are now required to produce homoeopathic remedies under very strict control and regulations laid down by the Medicines Act. One of the problems is that every potency of every remedy must be registered. Certain problems also arise when known toxic substances are prescribed over the counter in the chemist's shop direct to patients. This is perfectly safe in the higher dilutions but at the low dilution (below 10^{-12}) there is the possibility of toxic side-effects, and regulations to control this are at present under discussion.

At approximately 24 × or 12C the solution should theoretically contain no molecules of the original substance. In practice, however, these 'potencies' still have an action, and are still specific in their symptomatology to the original substance. As yet there is no known explanation for this continued activity, but it seems that succussion is vital at each stage. Simple dilutions do not have the same effect. Research has been done which demonstrates activity in these solutions in the field of enzymes, plant growth, and physiological preparations. Some of these experiments are discussed in more detail later in this chapter. No explanation of why this activity is present has so far been forthcoming, nor of why the succussion is important in their preparation. It may well be that the action is not a purely pharmacological one in the higher dilutions, but some other form of energy. This whole field urgently requires research from experts in the sciences, because it has implications much wider than the use of homoeopathic remedies.

Practical prescribing

The remedies are prescribed in tincture given by mouth as drops (e.g. *Crataegus* in heart conditions) or in tablets, pills or granules. These have a common base of sucrose or lactose and the liquid potency is added to a bottle of these at whatever stage is required. Commonly used potencies are 6 ×, 12C, 30C, 200C, 1M, 10M. All remedies are available on NHS prescription and the doctor should write the name of the remedy, the potency, and the form (tablet, granules) and the number of tablets. A convenient pack is a 7-g vial which contains about 56 tablets, approximately a month's supply at two per day. The 6 × potencies are often given in this way. In acute prescribing a tablet should be given 2-hourly initially and then 4-hourly after the first day, stopping on improvement. In a very acute case tablets can be given every 5–10 minutes. A potency of 30C is a useful one for beginners and can be used for a patient of any age and in both acute and chronic prescribing. Many doctors in the UK use the Kentian method of prescribing a single remedy and in chronic cases only three doses are given 4-hourly, and the effect of the remedy is allowed to run for some weeks before repetition.

Sample prescription:

> ARNICA 30C
> 7 g
> One tablet 4-hourly until improvement.
>
> SULPHUR 6 ×
> 7 g
> One tablet twice daily.

Remedies are also available as creams or ointments, e.g. Burn ointment, Hypericum ointment.

Manufacturers now produce a series of simple home or first-aid remedies, and these are often seen in health food shops or pharmacies. Some of these are mixtures of several remedies with labels 'Hay fever pills' or 'Travel sickness pills'. These are often quite effective in simple ailments. Some doctors are, however, now concerned at the ease with which patients can purchase higher potencies of wide-ranging deep-acting remedies. If a patient takes a 30C tablet of a remedy like *Sepia* or *Natrum mur.* twice daily for weeks on end, she will often develop 'proving' symptoms, i.e. the very symptoms she is trying to cure. Improvement will not occur until she stops taking the remedy. There is a need to tighten legislation in this field.

In Germany and France and some other European countries the use of mixtures of low-potency remedies or tinctures is widespread. Several remedies are included in these mixtures and they are prescribed on a pathological basis, e.g. for liver or gall bladder complaints, for fever, for rheumatism, not on a full individualising case history. This certainly makes for easier prescribing by a doctor trained in conventional medicine, but to those trained in selecting a single remedy for an individual patient, based on the modalities and patient reactions, the use of complex mixtures seems to negate the very principle of selection of a similar remedy. The use of a single remedy based on the patient's total symptom picture was the method advocated by Hahnemann and Kent, the latter often using very high potencies. To select an accurate remedy in this way requires a detailed case history and much study. This may be a deterrent to a new doctor trying to prescribe homoeopathy, but if correctly chosen the effect will be wide ranging and prolonged.

Similarly, special 'nosode complexes' are also available and these are used to overcome the effect of toxins within the body. These may be the result of hereditary illness or of acquired illness due to bacterial or viral infections, or from the effects of environmental pollution or chemicals in food sprays. Some doctors now believe that certain chronic illnesses are a result of these toxins, and preparations made from discharges during illness (e.g. in the case of measles), or from bacteria, viruses, chemicals and allergens, are used to treat the after-effects of such illness. These are either single nosodes from a specific organism or toxin, or complexes containing a mixture. Further information on mixed homoeopathic remedies can be obtained in English from Noma Ltd, P.O. Box 80, Southampton.

If a patient has never been well since measles, a dose of *Morbillinum* would be given to start with, or if rheumatic symptoms followed recurring streptococcal infections, *Streptococcin* might be prescribed. A strong family history of tuberculosis would indicate the need for *Tuberculinum* in the child with asthma or recurring chest infections. A nosode remedy will not necessarily effect a cure on its own, but is often a good start to following prescriptions based on the patient's symptom picture.

The place of homoeopathy in clinical practice

Homoeopathy should be regarded as a complement to conventional therapeutics, and to other forms of therapy, and not as a complete substitute. With the tremendous pace of therapeutic advances, deeper understanding of the causes of certain diseases, the application of preventive medicine and the role of the modern biochemist, geneticist, anaesthetist and surgeon, there are some fields in which homoeopathy has little or no part to play. A sound knowledge of clinical medicine and diagnosis is essential in order to select the best therapy for the patient. Nevertheless, there is still a valuable place for homoeopathic prescribing before and after operations, in injuries, in infections and in many other common illnesses which present problems difficult to cure with conventional treatment.

As already mentioned, in deficiencies or overwhelming infection conventional drugs are essential, but homoeopathy can play a supporting role. In degenerative conditions and certain neurological diseases such as motor neuron disease, dystrophies, multiple sclerosis and Parkinson's disease, results with homoeopathic treatment are on the whole disappointing, although occasional unexpected improvements do occur. In the treatment of cancer some surprising results have been claimed. In the majority of these cases homoeopathy has a supportive role. Alleviation of pain and fear can often be considerable, and although the ultimate prognosis and life span may not be greatly changed, these patients can often be kept more comfortable and alert, with a minimum of analgesia and sedation.

What then can homoeopathy offer?

First aid and injury

Aconite is prescribed where there is fright, shock or chill, in which there is tremor, palpitation, hyperventilation with tightness of the chest and marked fear. It can be given repeatedly every 5–10 minutes both to the patient and to others present following an accident.

Arnica is indicated in an injury with bruising and soreness, falls, sprains, head injury. It will often prevent bruising or help it to resolve. It is also useful after operations, and is given every 15 minutes.

Rhus. tox. for the effects of strains where the muscle stiffness and aching are temporarily relieved by movement, and worse at rest. Also useful in rheumatic pains which are worse in the morning and improve on moving about.

Hypericum for nerve injuries, crushed finger, painful animal bites or lacerations. Along with *Arnica* it will often relieve pain.

Ledum is useful in puncture wounds and insect bites, but patients with deep potentially septic wounds should have tetanus immunisation.

In burns a special homoeopathic burn ointment is most effective in relieving pain and promoting healing, and *Cantharis* potency given by mouth is also of value.

Calendula tincture or ointment (Marigold) is excellent for local dressing of wounds and cuts, and in skin disorders.

Acute infections, respiratory and gastrointestinal illness

In acute homoeopathic prescribing careful observation of the patient plays an important part in selecting the correct remedy. The diagnosis will depend on a quick history, and clinical examination of the throat, lungs, abdomen, ears and urine, or the presence of a rash in infectious disease. The diagnosis is still important to a homoeopathic physician, but selection of the remedy requires further elucidation. Is the child hot and flushed, pale, dry or sweaty? Does he throw off the bedclothes or is he wrapped up or under the blankets? Is he thirsty or not, in spite of high fever? Does he lie still and resent being disturbed, crying out if touched, or is he restless, anxious, wanting reassurance and touch? Is he delirious? Is a pain better or worse from pressure, movement or warmth? What is the character of his cough—dry, tickly, loose, barking, spasmodic? When does it get worse—with cold air or talking, during the night at a specific hour? What is the stool or vomit like in colour and consistency?

To the average doctor this may seem largely irrelevant, but to a homoeopathic physician these characteristics (or *modalities*) will help him to select one remedy from another. In a case of measles the rash may be slow to develop, the cough may be dry and sore, the child thirsty with headache, white dry tongue and irritable if disturbed. *Bryonia* would be indicated here. Or he may be weepy, wanting attention, with sore eyes, loose cough and lack of thirst in spite of fever. *Pulsatilla* will soon clear up his illness.

There are those who say that with antibiotics there is little need for homoeopathy, but many acute illnesses are viral and conventional medicine has only symptomatic palliation to offer. A well-chosen homoeopathic remedy selected for an individual patient's symptom picture will stimulate his reaction to his illness with rapid recovery, fewer complications and no side-effects or allergy.

Useful acute remedies

Sore throats, otitis media, chill and early respiratory infections		Aconite Belladonna Hepar sulph. Mercurius sol.
Infectious fevers	Measles	Pulsatilla Bryonia Sulphur
	Chickenpox	Antimonium tart.
	Whooping cough	Drosera
Pneumonia and bronchitis (antibiotics may be indicated in some patients)		Bryonia Phosphorus Pulsatilla Antimonium tart. Kali carb.
Acute diarrhoea and vomiting		Arsenicum alb.
Dyspepsia and peptic ulcer		Nux vomica Phosphorus Graphites Argentum nit.

To prescribe for acute illness with homoeopathy only requires knowledge of about 20 common remedies, with their characteristic pictures and distinguishing features, and the ability to see a similar picture in the individual patient. It cannot be emphasised too strongly that selection of the correct remedy is vital and routine prescribing of *Belladonna*, for example, in all fevers or sore throats, will only help some patients. Nevertheless, a rapid cure of acute illness will do more to convince the physician of the effectiveness of homoeopathy than any number of clinical trials. The use of *Arnica* in injury and bruising has converted more sceptics than almost any other remedy.

Chronic disease

Many common chronic illnesses present problems to the general practitioner in their management and treatment. Either the patient fails to respond to drugs or the side-effects make it more and more difficult to cope with the symptoms. A large number of such cases come to homoeopathic doctors or are referred as a last resort.

In prescribing for chronic illness with homoeopathy we must approach the patient in a slightly different way than is our custom in conventional medicine.

History taking

The basic history taking of the present, past and family history is the same but the homoeopathic doctor is particularly interested in the onset of illness, even many years previously. Did it start after a fall or injury, following a fright, anger or a profound emotional experience, loss of a loved one, a broken engagement, or is there some deep-seated resentment smouldering on and causing ill-health? The importance of these factors is not just from a psychological point of view, but because there are remedies like *Arnica, Aconite, Opium, Colocynth, Ignatia* or *Staphisagria* which help patients to overcome these original sources of disturbance which have led to their present complaints. In the case of the past or family history, a strong history of tuberculosis or cancer might indicate the need for a tissue preparation nosode like *Tuberculinum* or *Carcinosin*. An allergic family history is of course important in any patient with asthma, eczema or rhinitis.

The complaint and present history

This will also require more elucidation than is usually necessary in basic diagnosis. Mention has already been made of modalities (factors which qualify a symptom) and in chronic disease these can be of great importance. The pain and stiffness of a rheumatoid arthritis may be modified either better or worse from rest, movement, damp, frost, cold, heat, sea air or thunder. There may be a time aggravation: always worse on rising or in bed at night. The character of the pain may be significant. These modalities will not usually alter the accuracy of the diagnosis, but they will profoundly affect the selection of one homoeopathic remedy from another.

Study of the patient

Having had a clinical diagnosis from the history, examination and investigations, and having ascertained the modalities of the presenting symptoms, the physician must then study the patient as a whole and as an individual with a particular reaction to his illness.

General reaction

What are his or her general physical and emotional reactions as a person to the evironment and have they changed with the illness? Is he a hot or cold person—worse or better in the hot sun or a hot room? Does he sweat unduly on his head, hands or feet?

Food likings

Has he any strong food cravings or dislike for sweet food, salt, vinegar, fat, eggs, milk or marked thirst for hot or cold drinks?

Sleep

What is his sleep pattern? Does he sleep in one position—on his face or back, or on one side? Does this position affect his symptoms, his asthma, headache, cough or pain? Does he dream a lot?

Menses

Is there much aggravation of symptoms or general well-being in relation to the menstrual period—before, during or after it?

Emotional symptoms

We then come to study the emotional make-up of the patient. Is he excessively tidy, and upset by disorder or mess, or is he untidy in appearance or habits, tending to fall over things or knock articles down? Is he a placid, unruffled person or extremely irritable and impatient or constantly hurried? Is he emotional and weepy, and if so is this helped or made worse by sympathy? Is he sensitive to noise, or smells or touch, or startled easily? What fears does he have—of the dark, being alone, of death, of heights, thunder, shut in places like lifts or crowds? Is he aggressive and forceful or shy and timid, lacking confidence, indecisive? Is he a constant worrier, anticipating events with an anxious appearance? Is there resentment, bitterness, anger, grief, jealousy or suspicion? Is he an extrovert, fond of people, of art, music, drama, or a reticent, bottled up, reserved type of personality?

Although people may have a basic personality and reaction to events, to others, and to illness, what is important in homoeopathic prescribing is a change from the normal as a result of the illness: a normally placid individual who becomes extremely angry, anxious, frightened or weepy; a sociable, bright, lively girl who becomes withdrawn, resentful and depressed. These changes would indicate the need for a remedy. In the course of this discussion and observation some sexual or marital problem may be brought to the surface, and the patient may feel a relief at being able to express this to someone.

Relevance of in-depth case taking

You may well be asking why all this is of any relevance in a case of asthma or migraine or arthritis. Surely this is just psycho-analysis and best left to the psychiatrist? If time allows or can be made to allow, an in-depth discussion of this kind in any practice situation may reveal some extraordinary underlying factors which can be helped, whether one is practising homoeopathy or not. But in homoeopathic prescribing in a chronic case much of this will be very relevant in selecting a remedy for that patient as a whole.

This approach to the chronic problem, taking into account the past and family history, the onset of the illness and then a study of that individual in terms of reactions to the illness, temperature, food, sleep, menstrual period and emotional symptoms as well as the modalities of the complaint itself, will enable the skilled practitioner to select a remedy from the materia medica which matches an appreciable number of the patient's symptoms. He can then prescribe it in potentised form. A single remedy covering a wide number of symptoms is always best. The patient will react to the administration of this remedy and in so doing his symptoms and signs will often clear up completely. In some instances symptoms he has never mentioned will also disappear, and above all his sense of well-being will return. This latter sense is often a good indication that the remedy is helping even before the local symptoms improve. A patient will say, 'I feel better than I have for 2 years'.

Although selection of a single remedy is emphasised, in chronic illness it may be necessary to repeat the same remedy at intervals depending on the response. It may also be necessary to follow one remedy with another: if symptoms change and in difficult chronic cases like severe arthritis, chronic bronchitis or psoriasis, ongoing treatment is required and response will be slow and in some cases only palliative. The selection of a remedy based on the total symptom picture is known as constitutional prescribing.

Types of patient

The concept of constitutional prescribing to promote well-being and better health and to reduce the relapse rate in recurring coughs, migraine, asthma or rheumatism can be enlarged still further by an understanding of patient types. These are described vividly by Margaret Tyler in her *Homoeopathic Drug Pictures*.

Arsenicum patients are often immaculate in their dress, with clean collar and shoes, and groomed hair. They keep their house or garden perfect and their belongings neat and orderly. The *Arsenicum* is also a person who is chilly, restless and full of fears.

Sulphur types are often hot, untidy, prone to theorise about their illness and are either stout, florid and cheerful or stooped and introspective. They frequently suffer from skin complaints.

Phosphorus patients are usually slender with dark eyes and hair, or freckles and red hair. Their eyelashes are long and they are sensitive, attractive, vivacious people with fears and a need for affection and physical touch—often artistic and musical.

Pulsatilla children are frequently fair, plump, tearful and jealous, wanting attention and often shy. They are sensitive to hot atmosphere and upset by rich food and suffer from catarrh, colds and coughs.

Silica children, on the other hand, are very chilly with cold hands and sweaty feet, very timid, lacking confidence, liable to septic spots and cuts.

Lycopodium patients are usually intellectual, and capable, often lawyers, accountants or doctors. They worry excessively and anticipate events, having an anxious frown and often suffer from dyspepsia or an ulcer.

The housewife who is tired, irritable, weepy and has lost interest in her home and family will often respond to *Sepia*.

Calcarea carb. suits pale, overweight, flabby children who are slow to develop, fearful and sensitive, and suffer from nightmares. These children have large tonsils and glands, frequent colds and catarrh.

These few examples may help to illustrate that by observation of the patient's appearance and mannerisms, as well as a full history previously described, we can often select a suitable constitutional remedy.

What types of chronic illness do homoeopathic doctors treat?

Skin conditions

Eczema, psoriasis or dermatitis. Here the aim is to treat the patient not just his skin. He may require diet to eliminate certain foods like dairy produce, coffee, chocolate, wheat, red meat or citrus fruits, and he may require local applications, occasionally steroid ointments, but preferably just bland emollients. The homoeopathic treatment will be by mouth, selecting the remedy as described not just on the skin appearance, but on the patient's total symptom picture.

Allergic conditions

Asthma, hay fever, migraine, urticaria and again eczema. It is better to treat conditions like asthma or migraine between attacks using the patient's constitutional remedy, although there are also remedies useful during the acute attack. Inhalers or bronchodilating drugs or even steroids may need to be prescribed as well in severe cases. Conditions like hay fever or allergy to house dust, animals, moulds or pollen require preventive measures to reduce exposure to the allergen, but prescribing a special vaccine (or nosode) for the specific sensitivity is often very effective. A recent pilot study using a homoeopathic potency of grass and pollen for hay fever, compared on a double-blind basis with placebo, showed a significant reduction in the hay fever symptoms (Reilly, 1983). House dust and dog and cat hair are also used in this way. Diet may again be extremely important, excluding certain allergic foods.

Rheumatism and arthritis

A great many patients come to all forms of alternative therapy with this group of diseases. Early cases, or those with minimal joint involvement, can be cured. Advanced cases of rheumatoid arthritis or osteoarthritis can be alleviated, but may require additional conventional drugs. Many patients are just unable to tolerate these drugs and may well respond to homoeopathy. The patient's well-being and ability to cope with the disease are often markedly improved, and some relief of pain and stiffness obtained.

Respiratory disease

Recurring tonsillitis and coughs in children are often treated with repeated courses of antibiotics. While these may in some instances clear up the acute illness, relapse is common.

Homoeopathic remedies can be used in the acute stage with excellent response, but it is also possible to treat the child on a regular long-term basis with remedies suited to the individual child—the constitutional remedy, taking into account the general reactions to environment and food and the personality of the child, as already described. *Calcarea carb., Pulsatilla, Phosphorus, Silica* and *Sulphur* and *Tuberculinum* are often used in this way. The child's general health will improve, his appetite increase, his temperament often adjust and his tendency to sore throats and coughs steadily disappear. This is a most rewarding field for prescribing.

Asthma is treated in both the acute and chronic stages as mentioned. Patients with chronic bronchitis can be helped by low-potency (6 ×) prescribing over long periods and by giving a constitutional remedy at intervals. They often need fewer antibiotics and are able to lead a more normal life.

Gastrointestinal disease

Mention has been made of some acute remedies, but conditions like peptic ulcer, hiatus hernia, irritable bowel syndrome, colitis, gall-bladder inflammation, chronic constipation and haemorrhoids will all respond to remedies based on both local and general symptoms. Needless to say, full clinical, laboratory, and radiological investigation should always be done, and surgery may be indicated.

Headaches

These present regularly in the surgery and a high proportion will be due to migraine or stress and anxiety. Here the underlying causes may be most important and a case-taking procedure as described will often uncover family or business reasons for the tension, as well as suggesting a remedy based on the emotional symptoms. Acute headache is treated by a remedy selected mainly on the modalities, type of pain and factors which modify it, with any marked mental symptoms, irritability, fear, desire for or aversion to company. In the chronic case a deeper understanding of the patient's personality will be more valuable in choosing a remedy.

Genitourinary conditions

The presence of calculi, fibroids or an ovarian cyst may require a surgical opinion, and some cases of cystitis or vaginal discharge may need antibiotics or antifungal drugs. If symptoms of frequency and pain are acute, remedies like *Cantharis* or *Causticum* will greatly relieve these. Patients with recurring bladder infections can be a problem, where repeated courses of antibiotic only produce temporary relief. Here the homoeopathic approach to the patient's total symptomatology will often reduce the incidence of attacks and sometimes eradicate them entirely. The prescription of remedies like *Sepia, Thuja, Staphisagria* or *Sycotic co.* will depend on a full case taking and not just the patient's bladder symptoms. Renal colic will often respond to *Berberis, Colocynth* or *Magnesia phos*. Leucorrhoea which fails to respond to the usual creams and pessaries may clear up with remedies based on local modalities, such as *Kreosotum* (extremely acrid, burning discharge) or *Mercurius* (very offensive).

Disturbances of the menstrual period can be helped by remedies—*Magnesia phos., Colocynth, Natrum mur.*, or *Caulophyllum* for dysmenorrhoea. Irregularities of the period or profuse periods respond to constitutional prescribing. Premenstrual tension and symptoms of the menopause require *Lachesis, Sepia, Natrum mur., Cimicifuga* or *Staphisagria*.

Cardiovascular disease

In gross cardiac failure or severe hypertension, conventional drugs are usually necessary, but homoeopathy can relieve symptoms of ischaemia, improve cardiac output, reduce irregularities of rhythm, and control certain cases of hypertension, without the problem of side-effects often encountered when using antihypertensive drugs.

Crataegus in tincture is helpful in cardiac muscle weakness or raised blood pressure. In collapsed patients with weak pulse, cold extremities, sweating and gasping for air, *Carbo veg.* can produce a dramatic response within a few minutes; and in the rattling respiration of left heart failure, *Antimonium tart.* is equally rapid in its action. Patients with intermittent claudication can increase their walking considerably with prescription of *Cuprum met.* (a cramp remedy) or *Calcarea carb. Cactus* and *Lachesis* help angina.

Psychosomatic illness and anxiety states

The percentage of patients in this group in the average general practitioner's surgery must be 60–70%. Prescribing of tranquillisers and antidepressants is now a major problem, and stopping them is even more difficult. If adequate time were available for sympathetic discussion and airing of problems, many patients could be helped without the need for tablets. There are those who argue that the homoeopathic doctor, by virtue of his casetaking procedure, particularly the study of the family and social history and the emphasis on the emotional reactions of the patient, is really obtaining a therapeutic response in this way irrespective of what remedy he prescribes. There is no denying that this approach plays an important role, but experience does suggest that certain major remedies prescribed on the total symptom picture and with particular emphasis on the mental symptoms like fear, jealousy, resentment, grief, anger can dramatically improve the well-being of some patients, enabling them to cope better with their problems, even when they cannot be removed.

The tired, irritable, weepy housewife will often become much happier and more interested in her home after a dose of *Sepia*. The intellectual, worried businessman with digestive upsets responds very well to *Lycopodium*. The girl with a broken love affair or the woman who has never been able to cry since her husband or mother died will often unwind, weep and feel much better able to face life after *Natrum mur*. Severe depression and psychotic states are extremely difficult to treat with homoeopathy and usually need skilled psychiatric care.

Research

Failure of homoeopathic doctors to produce adequate 'scientific' evidence for the action of their remedies has always been used as an argument against the value of this therapy. This lack of evidence is frankly acknowledged by those who practise it, although many hundreds of patients will vouch for its efficacy in their particular illness. There are two main lines of research which require study. First, is it possible to demonstrate an active agent by modern laboratory techniques in a homoeopathic 'potency' of high dilution, which theoretically should contain none of the original substance? Second, is there any evidence of remedy action in clinical controlled trails?

Laboratory research

The difficulty here is to decide what to look for. Is the homoeopathic action due to a pharmacological effect on body tissues or the immune mechanism, or is it some form of electrophysical energy which affects the body's electrical field? Could its action be due to stimulation of naturally occurring endorphins or enkephalins as occurs in acupuncture? At present we do not know. Various research experiments have been carried out on plants, animals and enzymes which have demonstrated activity in a potentised solution.

Boyd (1954) demonstrated the effects of 30C potencies of mercuric chloride on a starch–diastase preparation which showed clear evidence of stimulation or inhibition as compared with controls under very rigid laboratory conditions. He also produced similar effects on perfused frog hearts. Unfortunately this work has never been repeated.

Netien *et al.* (1966) carried out experiments on the growth of plants which were poisoned with copper sulphate and then treated with potencies of copper sulphate (15C). Clear evidence of the activity of the potencies in reversing this poison was demonstrated.

Cier *et al.* (1967) published papers in which mice were given a 9C potency of *Alloxan* and then injections of *Alloxan*. The diabetogenic effect of the injections was greatly modified by the potency.

Raynor *et al.* (1981, 1983) have demonstrated in several papers the action of potencies on the growth of wheat coleoptiles and on yeast in dilutions up to 10^{-24}, studying the effects of succussion in the preparation of these dilutions on similar models. They postulate that succussion may cause molecular changes within the water–alcohol solvent, with alterations in the electrical field of the chains of molecules. Thus solvent continuity may be perpetuated by the impress made on the solvent, allowing the specificity of the original remedy to exist at high dilutions.

Moss *et al.* (1982) have demonstrated that low-potency remedies in the range 2×10^{-10} to 10^{-16} g/ml dilution of the source material are capable of modifying the movement of human leucocytes and guinea-pig macrophages in vitro, under controlled laboratory conditions.

Jean Kollerstrom (1982), in a paper entitled 'Basic scientific research into the "low-dose effect"', summarises some of this research and makes some pertinent observations about the difficulty of repeating such experiments.

Theories of so-called energy medicine have been explored by Vithoulkas (1978). Modern physics now looks at relationships and interactions in which parts are themselves changed in some way as a result of interacting one with another. Field theory, quantum theory, and relativity theory are being reflected in biological science in research into electrodynamic fields of the human body.

Instruments are now capable of measuring the electromagnetic field of the body (Burr, 1972). Kirlian photography is a technique whereby the electromagnetic field can be directly visualised.

Any substance can affect the human organism in one of two ways: by direct chemical action, or through interaction of electromagnetic fields, if the frequencies are close enough to resonate. A homoeopathic remedy may have a resonant frequency which can interact with the frequency produced by the body tissues, and thereby bring about a state of equilibrium, where this has been disturbed in illness.

Biologically active substances are capable of acting chemically on the tissues of the body, depending on the degree of susceptibility or affinity of the substance, but this tends to be a temporary effect. To obtain curative results, it is necessary to increase the intensity of the electromagnetic field of the substance. This may be possible by potentisation (dilution with succussion). The force of the electromagnetic field of the original substance is transferred to the solvent molecules, yet without changing the resonant frequency.

Alternative therapies are couched in terms of biological energy and therefore tend to have an intrinsically dynamic view of the body with concepts of energy flow. Conventional medicine has a mechanistic view of the body and concentrates more and more on individual parts. In homoeopathy all aspects of the patient's problem are seen in terms of their relatedness to each other, as in the world of modern physics, and the effect of the mind on the physical body is given much more emphasis.

Claims are now made that selection of a homoeopathic remedy by matching the frequencies of the patient's own field and the frequencies of the remedy is possible using bioenergetic regulatory techniques (Kenyon, 1983).

Clinical research

There is much evidence in homoeopathic literature of the effects of remedies on individual patients or a series of cases, but few properly controlled trials have been carried out.

Gibson *et. al.* (1978, 1980) carried out two series of controlled trials on rheumatoid arthritis. In the first of these, 41 patients were treated with high doses of salicylate and compared with a further 54 similar patients treated with homoeopathic remedies. Both groups were compared with 100 patients who received placebos. The patients who received homoeopathy improved more than those on salicylate, but criticism of this was based on the fact that the homoeopathic group was allowed to continue previous orthodox therapy while the salicylate group did not. Also, the patients in each group were seen by different doctors.

The second trial made a rigid comparison between one group of 23 patients on orthodox first-line anti-inflammatory treatment plus homoeopathy and a second group of 23 patients on orthodox first-line treatment plus an inert preparation. There was a significant improvement in subjective pain, articular index, stiffness and grip strength in those patients receiving homoeopathic remedies, and no significant change in the patients who received placebo. Both groups were seen by the same two physicians and the experiment was done under double-blind conditions.

A recent pilot study by Reilly (1983) on a group of hay fever patients, 11 of whom received a 30C potency of Pollen and Grass vaccine and 25 of whom received inert tablets in a 4-week study using a double-blind technique, showed both clinical and statistical confirmation of the effect of the potentised remedy as compared with placebo. A larger trial is planned for the summer of 1984.

Animal studies are also of interest and a recent article in *The Veterinary Record* (Day, 1984) describes a trial using *Caulophyllum* 30C on 10 farrowing sows in an intensive unit, a further 10 acting as controls. Prior to the trial the rate of stillbirth was around 20%, but after treatment twice weekly for 3 weeks before farrowing the percentage fell to 10% in the treatment group, remaining at 20.8% in the untreated group. When treatment of the whole herd of 130 sows was adopted the piglet mortality fell during the following 4 months to 2.6%. When *Caulophyllum* was stopped in the sixth month of the monitoring period, mortality rose steadily to 14.9% by the end of the eighth month. Treatment was then reinstated and in months 9 and 10 mortality again fell to 1.9%

Clinical trials in homoeopathy have always been difficult to design. Specific diseases may require different remedies depending on the individual's symptom picture, and it is therefore more difficult to plan a trial of one remedy against placebo or an orthodox drug. The type of trial described above is an exception. It is also necessary to decide what constitutes improvement in a particular illness. Assessment of conventional drugs in arthritis will use the parameters mentioned in Gibson's trial, but does not take into account the patient's well-being, the improvement in emotional state or attitude to his illness which may be equally important aspects of recovery or improvement. An attempt to study the effects of *Arnica* on postoperative pain in surgical patients brought out the considerable variations in individual patients' reactions and pain awareness. This even varied in different ethnic groups. So no two groups of patients were really comparable for drug and placebo effect.

Research is urgently required in both clinical and laboratory fields if homoeopathy is going to be accepted by the scientific medical field as a recognised alternative therapy in many common illnesses. Experts in physiology, biochemistry, immunology, psychology and clinical medicine must be encouraged to look seriously at homoeopathy, and considerable finance, at present unavailable, needs to be found.

Referrals

What patients should you as a general practitioner refer to a homoeopathic physician?

An outline has been given of the wide range of acute and chronic illnesses which can be helped by homoeopathy. Acute disease is best treated by the GP himself, and with a basic knowledge of a few acute remedies many common conditions can be satisfactorily cleared up, sometimes with the addition of an antibiotic as a second-line therapy if this is felt to be necessary. Accidents, injuries and infectious fevers are particularly rewarding.

In more chronic conditions it is unwise to attempt to treat everything which comes to the surgery with homoeopathy. Study a few remedies in depth and then wait until you see a clear prescribing picture in a patient which matches one of these. Do not be dismayed by some disappointing results—it is not usually because the remedy is inactive, but because our skill in selecting a suitable remedy is not adequate.

Patients may ask for referral to a homoeopath and most hospital clinics and many private physicians do prefer a letter, particularly if there is useful background information or investigation reports. Please do not refer only the 'last resort' patients who have had everything else, the neurotics and advanced neurological cases. Some of these may be helped but many will not respond to homoeopathy.

Allergic problems, recurring throat and chest infections in children, colitis and stomach disorders (provided they have been fully investigated), migraine, psoriasis, rheumatic conditions, certain gynaecological disorders, and patients with anxiety, depression or emotional upsets may all benefit from a homoeopathic approach.

As already stated, chronic conditions often require regular and prolonged prescribing to effect a cure, so do not expect a rapid result in every case. In acute disease, however, very rapid response will occur with the correct remedy, within hours or a day or two.

Sometimes, in chronic disease, symptoms may be exacerbated during the first week—the homoeopathic aggravation. This is due to the body's response to the stimulus of the remedy; the skin becomes more itchy, the joints more painful, even the emotions stirred up. This is usually a good sign of remedy response, and improvement will often follow.

Homoeopathic remedies do not have side-effects as we know them with orthodox drugs; they are safe to use in pregnancy, and will not poison the children, even if a whole bottle is eaten. They do not have long-term adverse effects, but too many remedies, given too frequently, especially in high potency, can cause quite profound disturbance and difficulty for another prescriber. It may be wise to stop all remedies for some weeks.

Lay homoeopathic practice

Because of the increasing demand for homoeopathy, a number of colleges have been started specifically to train homoeopathic practitioners who do not have a medical qualification. Some of these run very good courses in the principles and practice of homoeopathy and detailed study of the materia medica with particular emphasis on the totality of patients' symptoms and the matching of the similar remedy. They regard the medical pathological approach as a failure to see and treat the patient as a whole. Although they do teach some basic physiology and pathology, the lack of a full medical training may lead to errors in diagnosis, and failure to use certain conventional therapeutic methods which doctors feel are essential to good practice.

The Faculty of Homoeopathy has considerable reservations about the wisdom and safety of such practice.

Training in homoeopathy

The faculty organises short 2- and 3-day courses for doctors in London and Glasgow as well as seminars and discussion groups in other centres. These are designed to give a busy GP or hospital doctor the chance to learn basic homoeopathic skills to use in his own practice. Lectures and discussion and guidance in reading are given and doctors are encouraged to study for the Diploma of Membership (MFHom.). There is also a 6-month course at the Royal London Homoeopathic Hospital of lectures, ward rounds, discussion and case taking. Doctors are also encouraged to sit in at out-patients to see practical prescribing and follow-up of patients.

References

Boyd W. E. (1954). Biochemical and biological evidence of the activity of high potencies. *British Homoeopathic Journal*; 44:6.

Burr H. S. (1972). *The Fields of Life*. New York: Ballantine.

Cier A., Boirin J. *et al.* (1967). Experimental diabetes treated with infinitesimal doses of alloxan. *British Homoeopathic Journal*; 56:51.

Cook T. M. (1981). *Samuel Hahnemann. The Life and Work of the Founder*. Wellingborough: Thorsons.

Day C. E. I. (1984). Control of stillbirth in pigs using homoeopathy. *The Veterinary Record*; 114 (9):216.

Gibson R. G. Gibson S. L. M., MacNeil A. D., Gray G. H., Carson Dick W., Watson Buchanan W. (1978). Salicylates and homoeopathy in rheumatoid arthritis; preliminary observations. *British Journal of Clinical Pharmacology*; 6:391.

Gibson R.G., Gibson S. L. M., MacNeill A. D., Watson Buchanan W. (1980). Homoeopathic therapy in rheumatoid arthritis: evaluation by double-blind clinical therapeutic trial. *British Journal of Clinical Pharmacology*; 9:453–9.

Hahnemann S. (1982). *Organon of Medicine*, 6th edn. Translated by Kunzli J., Naude A., Pendleton P. London: Gollancz.

Jones R. L., Jenkins M. D. (1983). Comparison of wheat and yeast *in vitro* models for investigating homoeopathic medicines. *British Homoeopathic Journal*; 72:143–7.

Kenyon J. (1983). *Short Manual of Vegatest Method: Bioenergetic Regulatory Techniques*. Frankfurt: Vega-Griesharber.

Kollerstrom J. (1982). Basic scientific research into the 'low dose effect'. *British Homoeopathic Journal*; 71:41–7.

Moss V. A., Roberts J. A., Simpson K. (1982). The action of 'low potency' homoeopathic remedies on the movement of guinea-pig macrophages and human leucocytes. *British Homoeopathic Journal*; 71:48–61.

Netien G., Boiron J., Martin A. (1966). Copper sulphate and plant growth. *British Homoeopathic Journal*; 55:186.

Reilly D. (1983). Communication to the Midlands Homoeopathy Research Group Symposium.

Tyler M. L. (1942). *Homoeopathic Drug Pictures*. London: Homoeopathic Publishing Company.

Vithoulkas G. (1978). *The Science of Homoeopathy*, Vol. 1. Athens: Athens School of Homoeopathic Medicine.

Further reading

Blackie M. G. (1976). *The Patient not the Cure*. London: Macdonald & Jane's.

Boericke W. (1927). *Materia Medica with Repertory*, 9th edn. Revised by O. E. Boericke. New York: Boericke & Runyon.

Boyd H. W. (1981). *Introduction to Homoeopathic Medicine*. Beaconsfield: Beaconsfield Publishers.

Kent J. T. (1897). *Repertory of Homoeopathic Materia Medica*. Lancaster, Pa.: Examiner Printing Office.

Kent J. T. (1900). *Lectures on Homoeopathic Philosophy*. Lancaster, Pa.: Examiner Printing House.

Kent J. T. (1904). *Lectures on Homoeopathic Materia Medica*. Philadelphia: Boericke & Tafel.

Kenyon J. N. (Trans.) (1983). *Nosode Complexes*. Pascoe.

Kenyon J. N. (Trans.) (1983). *Similiaplexe*. Pascoe.

Pratt N. J. (1980). *Homoeopathic Prescribing*. Beaconsfield: Beaconsfield Publishers.

These books and the following booklets are available from The Faculty of Homoeopathy, 2 Powis Place, Great Ormond Street, London WC1N 3HT, from The British Homoeopathic Association, 27a Devonshire Street, London W1N 1RJ and from all major stockholding booksellers and homoeopathic pharmacists.

Gibson D. M. (n.d.) *Elements of Homoeopathy*. London: British Homoeopathic Association.

Gibson D. M. (1977). *First Aid Homoeopathy in Accidents and Ailments*, 6th edn. London: British Homoeopathic Association.

Jack R. A. F. (1980). *Introducing Homoeopathy into General Practice*.

Useful addresses

Faculty of Homoeopathy
The Royal London Homoeopathic Hospital
Great Ormond Street
London WC1N 3HR.
(Courses of postgraduate instruction, Associate Membership, faculty
library and secretariat.)

Scotish branch:
Glasgow Homoeopathic Hospital
1000 Great Western Road
Glasgow G12 ONR.
(Teaching courses and meetings.)

Midlands branch:
Dr R. A. F. Jack
The Limes
Lydiate Ash
Bromsgrove
Worcester B61 0QL.

Mossley Hill Hospital
Dr A. Ghosh
Homoeopathic Department
Park Avenue
Liverpool L18 9BU.

Bristol Homoeopathic Hospital
Dr J. S. Hughes Games
Cotham Road
Bristol BS6 6JU.

Tunbridge Wells Homoeopathic Hospital
Dr A. Clover
Church Road
Tunbridge Wells
Kent.

Chapter 5

Clinical ecology
J. Kenyon

Introduction

Clinical ecology is a discipline which applies the idea that
disease is wholly or partially caused by food and/or chemical
sensitivity. There has been increasing interest in these ideas in
the medical profession worldwide. Food and chemical sensitivity has, however, been recognised and used in a therapeutic
sense by naturopaths for many years. As a result, ecology at the
present time stands at the interface between conventional and
alternative medicine, much to the annoyance of many conventional doctors who are using ecology in their clinical work. The
clinical findings in ecological illness raise many unanswered
questions which have not and are not being faced by conventional doctors interested in this subject. To that extent
alternative medicine is able to adopt a more open-minded and
potentially more informative approach. As a consequence this
chapter is of a controversial nature. My aim is to give a broad
overview of ecology both from a conventional and alternative
standpoint, and to indicate a number of possible ways of
managing ecological illness.

History

The idea that allergy or sensitivity to certain foods can be a caus-
ative factor in disease is not new; Hippocrates was aware of
food reactions. The use of this concept in clinical medicine did
not begin till a number of American doctors, including Dr Albert
Rowe (a Californian doctor), revived it in the 1920s and 1930s
and invented the idea of an elimination diet which left out all

foods of a particular kind, such as grains or citrus fruits, to see if the patient's problem improved. Dr Rowe was able to tie up the disappearance of many chronic symptoms, such as headache, depression, rheumatism, irritable bowel syndrome, lack of energy and even, in some cases, epilepsy and multiple sclerosis, with the elimination of one or a number of foods. These remarkable clinical results naturally interested Dr Rowe's colleagues, and his work was further confirmed and extended by many other American doctors including such notable names as Rinkel, Randolph and Zeller. Double-blind test feedings were carried out and reported in the literature, as were correlations between conventional intradermal skin testing and the clinical diagnoses of food sensitivity. Many such references are contained in Rinkel *et al.*'s book, *Food Allergy* (1951), which introduced the idea of masked sensitivity in an attempt to explain the phenomenon of food reaction. This caused much controversy amongst conventional colleagues who considered that if an allergic reaction could not be demonstrated in the conventional sense, then food allergy did not exist.

Dr Randolph of Chicago extended the idea of ecology to include chemical sensitivity. (Randolph also introduced the 5-day fast at the beginning of food sensitivity investigation.)

Ecology began to attract the interest of doctors in the United Kingdom in the early 1970s and this was marked by the formation of the Clinical Ecology Group. Meanwhile, naturopaths and various doctors practising alternative medicine had been using the concept of food and chemical sensitivity since at least the turn of the century.

Definitions

It is of some importance to define food sensitivity more carefully and to identify those reactions which are truly allergic and those which are not. The assumption that food sensitivity implies true allergy has been one of the major obstacles to the acceptance of clinical ecology by conventional medicine. Therefore the argument has largely devolved into a semantic one between allergy and sensitivity which is proving fruitless in terms of elucidating the mechanism of action of food sensitivity as opposed to food allergy. It is proposed to classify food sensitivity along the lines adopted by the Royal College of Physicians report on *Food Intolerance and Food Aversion* (1984).

Food allergy

This is to be understood as a true allergic reaction in which there is accompanying evidence of an abnormal immunological reaction to the food.

Food sensitivity

This is a state in which there is no evidence of an abnormal immunological reaction. It can be divided into five groups as follows.

I Psychological reactions to food from various causes.

II Enzyme deficiencies, for example lactase deficiency.

III Pharmacological reactions to food, for example due to large amounts of chocolate (containing tyramine) or to drinking strong coffee (caffeine).

IV Food reactions due to a histamine-releasing effect in unsensitised individuals, for example caused by consumption of shellfish or strawberries.

V Irritant effect of foods on the gastrointestinal mucous membrane, especially when this is diseased. This occurs in certain individuals sensitive to wheat bran or to very spicy foods.

Three of these mechanisms need discussing further: psychological, enzyme deficiencies and pharmacological reactions.

Psychological reactions

Clinical ecology has become a haven for many patients whose problems are fundamentally psychological. It is perhaps unfortunate that one of the best-known lay books on ecology implies that most psychological problems are due to ecological causes (Mackarness, 1976, Ch.1). It requires a balanced view of both conventional medicine and ecology for any doctor to recognise psychological problems which are due to ecological causes and those which are truly psychological. In practice only a minority of psychological problems appear to have ecological causes. An overenthusiastic approach by the practitioner is often to the ultimate detriment of the patient as more and more extreme dietary measures are taken in order to convince both patient and doctor that the psychological problem has an ecological basis.

Enzyme deficiencies

The best example of food sensitivity due to lack of enzymes is lactase deficiency, of which there are two forms, congenital and acquired. The congenital type seems to be racial, being particularly common in oriental and negro populations (Haverberg *et al.*, 1980). The symptoms of hypolactasia are almost always abdominal and often mimic irritable bowel syndrome. Many other much rarer enzyme deficiencies are described, such as fructosaemia, galactosaemia and glucose-6-phosphate dehydrogenase deficiency, to name a few. The majority of these are diagnosed very early in life, if not during the neonatal period, and to that extent hardly fall within the realm of clinical ecology.

Pharmacological food reactions

A direct pharmacological effect of certain foods has been suggested as a cause for symptoms arising due to their consumption (Lessof, 1983). Some food additives, and particularly colourants, such as tartrazine, have been postulated as having a pharmacological mechanism (Moneret-Vautrin, 1983).

Prevalence of food sensitivity

The general assumption has been that the incidence of food, and indeed chemical, sensitivity is on the increase. Evidence for this is entirely conjectural and rests on clinical impression. Unfortunately there is no way of testing this supposition and therefore it is difficult to know what value to give to the varying estimates of prevalence found in the literature. For example, it has been suggested that between 0.3% and 20% of children suffer from, or have suffered from, symptoms caused by some form of dietary intolerance (Ogle and Bullock, 1977). Many of the wilder claims for the prevalence of food sensitivity arise from highly opinionated sources and are therefore difficult to believe. If, however, toxicity produced by environmental chemicals of various sorts (particularly pesticides, fungicides, weedkillers and hydrocarbon pollution) is accepted as being an underlying cause of food and chemical sensitivity, then it is entirely reasonable to assume that the incidence of ecological illness is on the increase.

Mechanisms of food sensitivity/allergy

Food allergy

This is an immunologically mediated reaction and is therefore easy to diagnose using conventional skin tests and immuno-globulin estimations, as described later in this chapter.

Food sensitivity

The mechanisms of action listed under definitions have been adequately described. The idea of masked sensitivity attempts to explain clinically food intolerance which is assumed to be due to one or a number of the mechanisms mentioned under definitions.

Allergy or sensitivity?

The question as to whether food and chemical reactions are truly allergic or not has been a point of argument between conventional allergists and ecologists. A number of food reactions are truly allergic phenomena with accompanying immunological changes such as raised IgE levels. However, most reactions to foods and chemicals are not truly allergic in nature, i.e. they do not yield positive skin tests and neither do they show appropriate immunological changes. It is therefore more correct to speak of sensitivity rather than allergy.

Masked sensitivity

One of the main criticisms levelled at the early clinical ecologists working in America was that there was no obvious reaction to the food while the patient was ill. This reaction only became obvious after the patient had fasted for at least 5 days and then had the foods reintroduced one by one (the so-called elimination diet). A clinical mechanism was therefore suggested which involved the idea that when the patient was ill the sensitivity was masked and only became unmasked after fasting. Following a 5-day fast, the patient is clinically in a so-called hyperacute state and usually reacts within a few minutes to the offending food. These reactions can be severe. After a few days the patient moves into a less sensitive state known as active sensitisation. This stage lasts a few weeks during which time the reactions are neither so marked nor so prolonged. After a period of weeks the patient then enters a stage of latent sensitisation during which reactions can be difficult to detect. Ultimately, after some months, the patient enters a state of tolerance when he is able to take the forbidden food on a rotation diet basis. If the food is taken more frequently than once every 3 days, then masked sensitivity occurs again with the reappearance of the old symptoms. This is illustrated in Fig. 5.1.

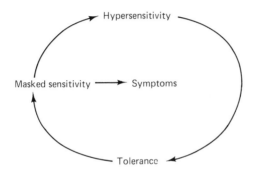

Fig. 5.1 The cycle of masked sensitivity and tolerance.

This explanation did nothing to satisfy the critics of the early American ecologists, but nevertheless remains a useful clinical idea on which to base management of the patient (Rinkel *et al.*, 1951, p. 30). If the patient is not able to tolerate the food again, perhaps because of an underlying enzyme deficiency, then his food sensitivity is classified as fixed. Most food sensitivities are temporary and the foods can be reintroduced after a sufficient period of avoidance. Mackarness (1980, p. 152) gives a useful analogy for visualising masked sensitivity. He suggests that the body is rather like a barrel. Usually we can cope with all foods and chemicals with which we are in regular contact. He suggests that these physical stresses can be visualised as water filling the barrel. In other words, most of us are healthy and can cope with most stresses (water) to which we are exposed. If we cannot cope with these environmental stresses, then the barrel overflows and symptoms result. This analogy has a number of important implications in that the problem can be looked at from decreasing the environmental stresses (sensitive foods and chemicals) or in terms of the patient himself (the barrel). In other words, if for any reason the patient is debilitated, then symptoms due to food sensitivities may occur on an intermittent basis. This is most commonly seen in women premenstrually. The clinical implication is that the body's normal immune defences do not function as well premenstrually as during the rest of the cycle.

The radiation theory

A number of clinical observations have led to the somewhat unconventional supposition by many ecologists that another, as yet undiscovered but important, mechanism is at work in food and chemical sensitivity (Lewith and Kenyon, in press). The implication is that sensitive foods or chemicals radiate in some as yet ill-understood manner and the patient reacts to this radiation. This idea has arisen due to phenomena seen when testing patients using the auricular cardiac reflex (ACR) or electrical testing (see later). A number of these patients develop symptoms during testing simply by having the substance placed near to them (when using the ACR) or in circuit with them (when using the Vegatest method for electrical testing), without in either case the substance having been in direct physical contact with the patient. This is a real phenomenon and is worthy of further investigation. It however remains the most controversial of the mechanisms of food and chemical sensitivity.

Regulation of immune response to food

It is interesting to consider why the immune system does not react to all ingested or inhaled substances. In order to do this it is useful to look at the mechanisms that allow tolerance to be acquired. Very few researchers have examined this problem, but it is clearly an interesting area as it may well elucidate some of the mechanisms underlying abnormal reactions to foods and chemicals (Ferguson *et al.*, 1983).

The intestinal immune system is composed of lymphoid follicles, mesenteric lymph nodes and secretory immunoglobulins (mainly IgA). It can respond in several different ways to orally administered antigen as both systemic and mucosal immune responses occur. Complex immunoregulatory networks mediated by helper and suppressor T cells have been found using rodents as experimental animals (Ferguson *et al.*, 1983).

Generally speaking, the feeding of antigen leads to mainly suppressor mechanisms in which suppressor T cells play a leading part in the Peyer's patches. Any inflammatory disease of the gastrointestinal tract is therefore of fundamental importance in precipitating a hypersensitive state.

The immunology of food sensitivity

A normal gastrointestinal mucosa is of major importance in enabling normal tolerance to ingested food (Jackson *et al.*, 1983). Immunological reactions to foods usually occur in the gut mucosa and submucosa. These are largely cell-mediated responses in which the T cells, both helper and suppressor, play a crucial role (Ferguson and Strobel, 1983). There is no available in-vitro test for food sensitivity.

The immunoglobulins, of which there are four main types (IgE, IgG, IgM and IgA), are also important in certain food sensitivity reactions. A food to which there is a true allergy triggers a reaction between complement (which is a complex series of substances) and an appropriate immunoglobulin, which as far as food is concerned, is likely to be an IgM or IgG. The end-result is to produce cell lysis, kinin release and, as a result, inflammation and symptoms relevant to the site at which these reactions are occurring. IgE is bound to mast cells and is present mainly in the skin, although there are small levels present in the serum. It is usually responsible for contact sensitivity and allergic manifestations such as urticaria. IgG is a serum antibody and is important (together with IgM) in many of the auto-immune diseases as well as in bacterial defence.

It has been suggested that deficiency of IgA predisposes to food allergy, as it removes the protective immunoglobulin coating of the gut mucosa, therefore causing increasing permeability of the gut to protein and other food antigens. It appears likely that in IgA-deficient individuals there may be deficient immunoregulation, centering around cell-mediated immunity; IgM and IgG class antibodies to many foods are present in the serum, although these do not necessarily produce classical food allergy. In other words, to assume that IgA deficiency can be the sole underlying cause of multiple food allergy would be simplistic, but it can be a factor.

Recently it has been found that in both healthy and food-allergic subjects circulating immune complexes are present shortly after ingestion of food. Interestingly, pretreatment with oral sodium cromoglycate relieves symptoms in those who were food allergic; it also reduces the amount of circulating immune complexes. The immunoglobulin present in these food-related immune complexes, in normal individuals, is predominantly IgA, whereas in food-allergic subjects they may also contain IgG and IgE and often bind complement. Therefore, in a normal immune response to food, with high levels of anti-food IgA antibodies, this leads to the production of harmless immune complexes which can be rapidly cleared from the serum. If the immune response is abnormal and, if for example IgG or IgE is contained in these complexes, then they cannot be cleared so easily and may produce symptoms. These abnormal immune complexes can therefore lead to stimulation of the inflammatory response, by triggering antigen-specific IgE-sensitised mast cells to release histamine. Also with complement activation, as a result of the formation of these immune complexes, chemotactic factors are released which attract neutrophils and mononuclear phagocytes which accentuate the inflammatory response (this is often localised, depending on where the sensitised mast cells are). This therefore means that looking for food-specific IgE in the serum is a sensible test for food allergy from the immunological point of view.

Immunological investigations in order to diagnose food sensitivity centre around the RAST (radio-allergosorbent test) which measures food-specific antibodies, specifically IgE. More recent tests are beginning to look at IgG and IgM levels. These will be discussed in more detail later.

Addiction and adaption

If the body is irritated regularly but intermittently, then it responds with a variety of different symptoms. If the irritation stops, then the symptoms often settle quickly, but should it continue, the body tends to adapt with very few attendant symptoms. In some cases the body's adaptive powers become exhausted and chronic symptoms ensue. This is the nub of Hans Selye's general adaption syndrome (Fig. 5.2).

Most sensitive food and chemicals can be viewed in this sense as chronic irritants. Hans Selye has described the above three stages (acute, chronic and maladaption) as the 'general adaption syndrome'. This principle can be applied to all biological

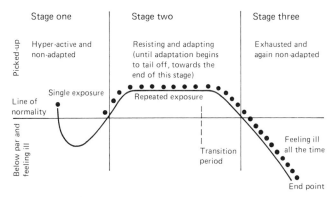

Fig. 5.2 Hans Selye's graph of general adaptation.

systems exposed to a hazardous environment and the consequent need to adapt. The conceptual models used to explain clinical ecology correspond closely to the general adaption syndrome. A simple explanation of the three stages can be made on the basis of a chronic physical irritant such as a badly fitting shoe. Stage one is a sore foot with a blister; if the shoe is discarded, the blister will heal. Stage two of the irritation is the formation of hard skin; if the shoe is worn only during part of the day, then no pain or other symptom occurs, but the skin hardens. The hard skin will become sore if the irritation is too forceful; consequently, even during the most adaptive stage, symptoms can result from excessive irritation. If the shoe continues to irritate, then the skin will eventually break down, and stage three is reached as the body fails to adapt.

Alcohol intake often falls into a similar pattern. Most people dislike alcohol initially. Certainly an excessive intake results in appropriate unpleasant symptoms. Prolonged excessive alcohol intake seems to have less effect and the patient seems to be able to imbibe increasing amounts with fewer obvious symptoms of drunkenness or hangover. This is the beginning of alcohol addiction. In due course the sufferer finds that he cannot start the day without regular alcohol. He then feels ill without alcohol and soon experiences symptoms if alcohol is withheld. Therefore the patient has reached stage three and this is accompanied by addiction to the sensitive food.

Sensitivity to foods or chemicals often follows a similar pattern. Similarly, withdrawal effects can be marked in many patients following elimination of a sensitive food which, by implication, they may be addicted to. This means that patient motivation is doubly important as often an addictive situation has to be dealt with.

Ecological illness

Ecological illness can be divided into two categories. The first is differentiated disease, that is recognised clinical diagnoses which can be due wholly or in part to an ecological cause. The second category is that of undifferentiated disease where an apparently unrelated group of symptoms is presented of which the underlying cause is ecological. Many illnesses have been found in some cases to have wholly or partial ecological bases. To that extent ecology is always worth a try in any illness which has not responded to any other approach.

Both categories of ecological disease have a surprisingly consistent list of associated symptoms. These are excessive fatigue, varying abdominal symptoms such as flatulence, disordered bowel habit, intermittent abdominal distension, to name but a few.

Diseases which can be due wholly or in part to food and/or chemical sensitivity are conveniently divided into those occurring in children and in adults.

Ecological disease in children

The following conditions have been found by most clinical ecologists in some cases to be wholly or partially ecologically based.

Behavioural problems

Sleep disturbance

A common cause of **sleep** disturbance in babies and young children is colic, which can act as a trigger for recurrent and persistent wakefulness. This can be due to food sensitivity, particularly to milk. Withdrawal of cow's milk from the diet of breast-feeding mothers has been shown to bring about an improvement in colic and therefore sleep in young babies (Jakobsson and Lindberg, 1978).

Hyperactivity

Marked sleep disturbance is a feature of hyperactivity as well as behavioural changes in that the child is often difficult to handle. The late Dr Ben Feingold, an American paediatrician, suggested that hyperactivity was an ecological problem and proposed that major causes were additives and colourings used in food. As a result he developed the Feingold diet (Leading article, 1979). In the experience of most ecologists, hyperactivity occurs with other more obvious food reactions such as migraine, disordered bowel habit, etc. Therefore a more specific dietary regime is often required in order to achieve a reasonable result. In many cases a hyperactive child is responding to a bad family situation which might have arisen from many causes, none of them ecological in any way. Therefore it is important for the doctor to be very sceptical of the application of an ecological approach to hyperactivity, but it is certainly a method worthy of trial.

Gastrointestinal symptoms

Persistent diarrhoea following gastroenteritis is commonly due to acquired food sensitivity resulting from mucosal damage from the original enteritis (Jackson *et al.*, 1983). This condition is relatively common in babies and young children, and responds well to an ecological approach.

Coeliac disease

This is caused by a sensitivity to gluten which damages the small intestinal mucosa. Gluten, a mixture of proteins, is a constituent of wheat, oats, rye and barley. The most common presentation is abnormal stools, vomiting, abdominal distension, irritability and failure to thrive. The treatment is a gluten-free diet and diagnosis is made conventionally by a small intestinal mucosal biopsy. Intolerance to gluten and coeliac disease are usually life-long, but transient gluten intolerance is observed regularly in ecological practice.

Constipation

Constipation is an uncommon complaint in young babies but is more prevalent in older children. It can arise as a result of psychological causes but an ecological approach should be considered.

ENT problems

The chronic catarrhal child

Children with recurrent chronic upper respiratory tract problems, and particularly 'glue ear', should be considered as having a possible ecological basis to their problems. Often these children respond gratifyingly to such an approach. It has been stated, however, that up to six upper respiratory tract infections can be expected per year in children between 4 and 7 years (*Food Intolerance and Food Aversion*, 1984, p. 12). It is difficult to know whether this indicates slightly below average health in all the child population or whether this really is the normality. Some ecologists have been impressed how, in families where a natural diet together with rain water is consumed regularly, the incidence of upper respiratory tract infections is much lower than the average. This is an interesting observation and one which ought to be looked into further.

Eczema

Food sensitivity and/or true allergy is an important cause of eczema and has been recognised as such within recent years (Abboton, 1982). Allergens such as the house dust mite have also been recognised more recently as being an important cause of contact sensitivity (Mitchell *et al.*, 1982). Desensitisation, homoeopathic remedies or using a Miller dilution (see page 201) for house dust mite often produces gratifying results in eczema.

Asthma

Asthma can in some cases have an ecological basis but is rarely sorted out completely using this approach alone. Generally speaking, the most successful approach in asthma within alternative medicine is to search for underlying causes using electrical measurement techniques and then to treat accordingly (Kenyon, in press). It has been claimed that tartrazine sensitivity can be a cause of asthma (Vedanthan *et al.*, 1977), and as tartrazine is chemically similar to aspirin, sensitivities to the two substances often occur together. Thus a diet low in salicylates* can be tried. Clinical studies of asthmatics with tartrazine sensitivity have, however, revealed widely varying results (Stenius and Lemola, 1976). Nevertheless, an ecological approach is certainly worth a try in childhood asthma.

Migraine

An ecological approach in childhood migraine often produces gratifying results. A recent trial carried out in Great Ormond Street Hospital for Sick Children, London (Egger *et al.*, 1983), demonstrated that almost 90% of children with migraine do have food sensitivities, and that their headaches respond to food exclusion; rechallenge with appropriate foods resulted in repeated headaches. The most commonly implicated food was milk followed by eggs, chocolate, orange, tea, wheat and artificial colouring coming lowest on the list. Experience in ecological practice shows that after 18 months to 2 years the sensitivity tends to disappear and the patient is then able to take the food again with some degree of regularity.

Other conditions

Other clinical problems have responded to an ecological approach, but the proportion of these patients relative to the total numbers having these illnesses is so small as not to be worthy of particular mention. However an interesting example is that epilepsy sometimes responds well to an ecological approach, but the percentage responding compared to total numbers with epilepsy would probably be less than 5%. Nevertheless, an ecological approach, as it is harmless, is well worth a try in these cases. Some ecologists would claim that it is worth a try in practically any illness. Providing this approach is used as an experiment, both on the part of the doctor and patient, then

---

* Salicylates are present in a number of fruits and vegetables such as cucumber, tomatoes, berries, apples and oranges. Many of the natural salicylates are stable and appear unchanged in food products such as preserves and wine. A number of synthetic salicylates are used to flavour sweets, ice cream, soft drinks and cake mixtures. The chemical similarity of salicylates with aspirin and tartrazine means that all these foods should be avoided in patients who are sensitive to tartrazine. This is an important cornerstone of the Feingold diet (Leading article, 1979).

there is no reason why it should not be carried out. It is very important to evaluate this properly by reintroduction of foods to see whether in fact the ecological approach in any condition for which it is tried is of some value. Otherwise restricted diets would be followed for longer than necessary with possible nutritional deficiencies. This is of major importance in children and therefore mitigates against a too enthusiastic application of very restricted diets in this age group.

Ecological illness in adults

Undifferentiated illness

Many ecologically based problems present as multiple symptomatology and it is tempting to diagnose these patients as being psychologically ill. The common symptoms in undifferentiated ecological illness include the following.

1. General malaise, often worse in the early morning and associated with difficulty in getting going. Often the patients complain that they wake up in the morning feeling as if they had not had a proper night's sleep.

2. Headache. This can be anything from a vague, unpleasant, 'heady' feeling to obvious migraine attacks.

3. Fluctuations in weight. Sometimes weight fluctuation may be as much as 4 or 5 kg in one day. In the extreme case patients have to have more than one wardrobe in order to dress for the appropriate time of day.

4. Abdominal distension and discomfort. Many patients complain of a feeling of distension, frequently worse after food. This symptom, like the three mentioned above, is not part of any conventional diagnosis and patients with this complaint often present having had a number of investigations, all of which were normal. Bowel disorders and excessive flatulence are common accompanying symptoms with abdominal distension.

5. Clouded mind. This is sometimes called 'brain fag' by the American clinical ecologists. Symptoms such as lack of concentration, forgetfulness, unexplained anxiety or mild depression may be associated with a whole series of vague physical complaints.

6. Excessive sweating, particularly at night.

7. Palpitations of unknown aetiology.

8. Rheumatic aches and pains with no clear diagnosis of arthritis on investigation.

9. Insomnia and excessive fatigue.

If five of these symptoms occur together, and particularly if they are of an intermittent nature, then this makes an underlying ecological cause a real possibility.

Obesity

The idea that food sensitivity could underlie some cases of obesity was first popularised by Dr Richard Mackarness (1961) in his book, *Eat Fat and Grow Thin*. The diets he recommends are based on avoiding foods to which people are commonly sensitive, such as wheat and milk. The book was a best seller, as were many books on weight loss. It puts forward an enthusiastic view of this approach to obesity, principally because the author was able to sort his own obesity problem out using this method. In practice it is successful in a small proportion of patients only, as with most of the other general approaches to weight loss.

Psychiatric disorders

The suggestion that anxiety and depression can be an ecological problem was made by Richard Mackarness (1976, Ch. 1) in his book, *Not all in the Mind*. Unfortunately, it is uncommon to find food sensitivity as a sole underlying cause in these patients. In other words, there are often accompanying symptoms which suggest that the food sensitivity is only part of the picture. In my own experience, ecology is a useful adjunct to treatment in psychiatric disorders but rarely succeeds as an exclusive approach.

Excessive sugar and junk food intake has recently been implicated within institutions such as prisons as an important cause of violent and aggressive behaviour by the inmates. Behaviour improves considerably if these foods are removed from the diet. In behaviour problems in general the beneficial effect of removing processed foods and any food with a high sugar content, particularly refined sugar, has been noted by many clinical ecologists.

Psychotic illness

There have been claims that schizophrenia is due to food sensitivity (Grant *et al.*, 1983), although this has not been confirmed (Dohan, 1966). The earlier paper implicated grains and there is a higher instance of schizophrenia in patients with coeliac disease, and peptides derived from gluten can be detected in the brain (Cooke and Holmes, 1983). The mechanism of action of food sensitivity in these cases has been surmised as one in which the sensitive food affects neurotransmitters and therefore produces abnormal behaviour. It is well known that certain food constituents can do this, i.e. high-carbohydrate low-protein meals elevate brain tryptophan which accelerates the synthesis of the neurotransmitter serotonin (Anderson, 1981). Unfortunately, the use of ecology in schizophrenia has been uniformly disappointing and I remain suspicious of some ecologists who claim 'cures' from a solely ecological approach in this disease.

Disseminated sclerosis

A number of patients with disseminated sclerosis have noted a marked improvement with an ecological approach. I have personally come across a number of such cases. My conclusion is that the diagnoses were mis-diagnoses in the first place and that in fact the patients were suffering from a bizarre collection of symptoms mimicking multiple sclerosis. It is nevertheless gratifying to be able to tell a patient that the diagnosis of multiple sclerosis was not correct, as implied above.

Migraine

There is little doubt that certain foods can play a part in precipitating some attacks of migraine in some sufferers. Claims that ecology plays a major role in the management of migraine should be looked at with some scepticism. Ecology is, however, a reasonable approach in these patients, although it must be recognised that about 30% of migraine sufferers respond at least temporarily to placebo and that stress is a major precipitant of migraine attacks. Therefore a sympathetic understanding by the doctor, whatever therapy he is using, will have some considerable effect on the incidence of attacks. In my own experience, migraine tends to be multifactorial in that stress and foods may be involved. Stress may produce immunological effects by altering the T lymphocyte population, therefore making the patient less immunologically competent at times of stress. Therefore at a time of low stress a food to which the patient is supposedly sensitive, such as chocolate, may not produce an attack, whereas if the patient is anxious and feeling low, then the chocolate may be enough to precipitate a major attack. An excellent review of the relationship of diet to migraine has been presented by Hanington (1983). In practice, the use of an ecological approach in adult migraine is not as successful as in children: the 90% alleviation rate seen in children is at least halved in adults.

Arthritis

It is a common observation amongst patients with both osteo- and rheumatoid arthritis that dietary changes can improve their condition. As to whether they can cure their problem or not is quite another question. These claims remain anecdotal and there is little evidence that could stand up to critical evaluation. Studies have been done using an ecological approach in cases of rheumatoid arthritis without any convincingly positive results (Skoldstam *et al.*, 1979; Walport *et al.*, 1983). The use of diets in arthritis has been popular amongst lay practitioners and a number of books designed for the arthritic sufferer enjoy continued high sales (Dong and Banks, 1976). In my experience, an ecological approach is certainly worth a try in cases of osteoarthritis where more than one joint is involved, and in all cases of rheumatoid arthritis. Monoarticular arthritis is rarely helped by a dietary approach. Patients with rheumatoid arthritis need to carry on food exclusion for considerably longer than those with osteoarthritis if they are going to note any improvement.

In my experience, even where an ecological approach has been dramatically effective, the patient has always needed a physical procedure such as acupuncture or manipulation in order to produce satisfactory pain relif. In summary, therefore, ecology is a useful adjunct to the treatment of rheumatoid and multiple osteoarthritis but is rarely a cure in its own right. The same observation applies to other autoimmune diseases such as ankylosing spondylitis, systemic lupus erythematosus, dermatomyositis and scleroderma.

Diseases of the digestive tract

Coeliac disease

This has been dealt with under the section on children (see page 189).

Irritable bowel syndrome

Irritable bowel syndrome has been successfully managed with diet. The foods most frequently involved are wheat, corn, dairy products, citrus fruits, tea and coffee (Hunter *et al.*, 1983). Double-blind challenge studies showed that reactions to food appear to be dose related and may take as long as 48 hours to develop. No truly food-allergic phenomena were found, such as raised serum IgE.

Crohn's disease

Exactly the same remarks apertaining to irritable bowel syndrome apply to Crohn's disease (Hunter *et al.*, 1983).

Chronic gastritis

An ecological approach can be useful in this problem and one study has shown a correlation between raised serum IgE levels and the implicated foods (Rosen *et al.*, 183).

Colitis

May cases of colitis respond well to an ecological approach. Soothill *et al.* (1983) reported complete success in treating colitis in infants. Similarly gratifying results can also be expected in adults. It is important to look for underlying causes in all colonic problems. Many of them have a primary psychological cause, and this particularly applies to irritable bowel syndrome. Like many illnesses which respond to an ecological approach, the food sensitivity is only an aspect of the problem. In many cases it may be an effect of the underlying problem rather than its cause. This must be borne in mind when treating ecological illness in general and gastrointestinal disease in particular.

Urticaria

Allergy is an important cause of urticaria but evidence of classical allergic phenomena may not always be present. Food additives are often implicated, particularly the aspirin-related ones such as tartrazine (Juhlin, 1981). The response to provocation tests is often variable, and changes in temperature can precipitate an attack. Sometimes urticaria is called a 'cold' or a 'hot' urticaria depending on which temperature change precipitates it. Exercise can also be a potentiating factor. Treatment of urticaria using an ecological approach is usually successful but is often laborious as ingested chemicals need to be considered and these can be very difficult to identify, let alone to eliminate.

Eczema

The same comments apply to adults as for the management of childhood eczema, but like many diseases in adult life, it is more difficult to cope with than in children. Contact dermatitis can be regarded as a form of eczema which responds well to the removal of the irritant, which is often metal containing nickel.

Irritable bladder

In some cases this can be due to a food or, more often, a chemical sensitivity. If this can be identified, then treatment is often successful.

Chronic candidal infections

Chronic vaginal thrush can, in some cases, be due to an ecological cause. Avoidance of sugar- and yeast-containing foods can be most beneficial in these cases as Candida itself is one of the yeast family. However, treatment with Nystatin preparations is still mandatory.

Enuresis

Enuresis is not an uncommon problem in adulthood but occurs more often in children. In some cases an ecological approach can be useful, and sensitivity to chemical additives is the most likely finding.

Other diseases

Epilepsy can, in a very few cases, respond to an ecological approach, as can many other diseases. I have seen cases of back pain, trigeminal neuralgia, temporomandibular joint syndrome, tinnitus (to name but a few) respond dramatically to an ecological approach and also to become worse on rechallenge with the implicated foods. These cases remain anachronistic considering the number of patients presenting with each of these problems.

Ecological diagnosis

The key to managing an ecological problem is clearly the identification of the offending foods and/or chemicals which are thought to be causing the patient's problem. To this end a number of diagnostic procedures have been developed which clearly divide into two sorts, conventional and unconventional.

Conventional methods

The most commonly accepted method of ecological diagnosis is the elimination diet technique (Rinkel *et al.*, 1951, pp. 113–234). Simply stated, the patient is put on a spring-water fast for a period of 5 days. If symptoms clear in this time, then it is assumed that the problem is an ecological one. If symptoms clear partially, then the inference is that the problem is only partially ecologically based. Some authorities allow the patient to have lamb and pears during the 5 days on the basis that these foods are rarely implicated in ecological illness (Mackarness, 1976, Ch. 8). The foods are then reintroduced one by one, with each meal consisting of one food only. After a 5-day fast it is assumed that the patient will be in a stage of hyperacute sensitisation (see Masked sensitivity). Generally speaking, the best practice is to introduce the rarely eaten foods first as these are unlikely to be the cause of the patient's problem and thus a more varied diet can be built up more quickly, as, if each new food tried gives no reaction, the patient is able to continue eating these foods while adding one new food per meal. Therefore each meal becomes a testing session. When the rarer foods have been tested, the more common ones are tested in a similar manner. These are most likely to be the foods implicated and in ecological practice those most commonly causing sensitivity reactions are, in order of frequency:

milk and dairy products
wheat
coffee
chocolate
eggs
citrus fruits
corn (maize)

If an oriental population is looked at, the list of foods would be different, with rice appearing towards the top of the list; similarly, if an American population is looked at, corn would have a higher position on the list. This illustrates the general rule that the foods to which the patient is most likely to be sensitive are those foods which are most commonly eaten. It also implies that food sensitivity is nearly always multiple and rarely involves one food alone. In the hyperacute sensitisation stage, following the 5-day fast, reactions to a food are usually clear and include symptoms which come on within 10 minutes or so after ingestion. There is usually an accompanying tachycardia with an increase in pulse rate of more than ten beats per minute as compared to the resting rate, although some authorities regard this as an unreliable sign (Rinkel *et al.*, 1951, p. 169). The end-result is a list of offending foods which the patient should then avoid.

There are many practical problems with elimination dieting. The most troublesome is patient motivation, as in practice very few patients are willing even to contemplate the 5-day fast, and are generaly even less able to carry out the laborious and introspective work necessary to build up a list of sensitive foods.

Most ecologists, when writing about the elimination diet technique, imply that it is a method which gives clear diagnostic pointers. In practice this is by no means always the case, as often the patient's symptoms may be so vague as to make it impossible to decide whether a particular food brings them on or not. This particularly applies to symptoms such as depression, lassitude or general irritability. Secondly, symptoms do not always come on within 10 minutes of oral challenge and in some cases can be delayed for as long as 48 hours. Generally speaking, this makes elimination dieting an unhelpful approach in all except the most clear-cut and obvious cases.

In-vitro tests

The semantic argument surrounding ecology has crystallised around testing techniques to demonstrate the presence of so-called food allergy or, more properly, food sensitivity. The most common criticism levelled at ecology by conventional allergists is the fact that conventional skin testing (so reliable for airborne allergens) is a relatively useless technique for ecological diagnosis. The correlation of positive skin tests with observable clinical reactions to sensitive foods has been rated at approximately 30% in terms of accuracy (Rinkel *et al.*, p. 145). This clearly makes conventional skin testing worse than useless for ecologial diagnosis. The most commonly accepted testing method used by conventional doctors (Keneny *et al.*, 1983) is the radio-allergosorbent test (RAST), although there is little clinical evidence that the findings from RAST (which measures specific IgE antibodies to foods) are relevant to the patient's clinical problem. In other words, the findings from RAST rarely produce a positive clinical result (Denman, 1983). One study found that a diet in patients with migraine based on avoidance of foods to which the patient had demonstrable serum antibodies was no more effective than a new diet based on avoidance of a random selection of foods (Freed, 1983). Conventional medicine, however, remains hellbent on perfecting in-vitro diagnostic methods, whereas in reality all the reactions occur in vivo (*Food Intolerance and Food Aversion*, 1984, p. 38).

Unorthodox methods

Cytotoxic testing

This is based on the observation that white blood cells of food-allergic patients undergo changes of varying severity when placed in the presence of concentrates of foods to which the patient is sensitive. In practice there are many problems with this test in that it is expensive (costing approximately £60 for a basic screen of commonly eaten foods) and also the results have been shown to be variable (Black, 1956). In one test a well-known British laboratory failed to obtain reproduceable results on duplicate blood samples taken from the same subject at the same time (Ferriman, 1983). From a clinical point of view, the findings on cytotoxic testing do generally produce a clinically useful result; they all show multiple food and chemical sensitivities in all patients. In many cases they are very difficult to interpret as so many foods and chemicals appear to be implicated in each patient.

Sublingual drop testing

Dropping solutions of foods in specific dilutions sublingually in patients who have just completed a 5-day fast is a useful and well-tried method for identifying foods which cause sensitivity (Miller, 1972). Symptoms of intolerance are generally provoked within a few minutes of the sublingual drop being placed in the patient's mouth. However, a number of trials have failed to discriminate between control materials and food extracts using the sublingual drop technique (Committee on Provocative Food Testing, 1973; Breneman *et al.*, 1974). Nevertheless, sublingual drop testing remains a practical procedure, the main drawback being that it is time consuming.

Intradermal skin testing

This technique involves the intradermal injection of small volumes of specific dilutions of specific foods or chemicals to which the patient is thought to be sensitive (Miller, 1972). The injection of a series of dilutions, by convention diluted in steps of 5 (i.e. dilution 1 is diluted 5 times, dilution 2, 25 times, etc.), produces interesting whealing responses as compared to conventional intradermal skin testing when concentrates are used. Associated clinical symptoms are often provoked as in sublingual drop testing. The most interesting finding is the absence of a whealing response on the injection of the concentrate, with a subsequent appearance of a positive whealing response on injection of a dilution of the same concentrate. This is a phenomenon for which there is no satisfactory explanation at the present time, but it nevertheless provides a useful and reliable diagnostic method for testing food and chemical sensitivity. This method has been the subject of highly prejudiced criticism by some conventional doctors (Barnetson and Lessof, 1983). Its main drawback is that it is very time consuming and a number of hours of testing are required in order to work through most of the common foods in any particular patient. In some highly sensitive patients the clinical reactions provoked by intradermal injection (as with sublingual drop testing) can be difficult if not impossible to switch off. Catastrophic anaphylactic reactions have not so far been reported using these techniques but they nevertheless remain a theoretical possibility.

The auricular cardiac reflex (ACR)

This is a clinical test which relies on a movement of the standing wave of the radial pulse in response to placing a sensitive food or chemical within the body's field (Kenyon, 1983). In skilled hands it is approximately 80% accurate, which is equal to the other unconventional diagnostic techniques mentioned so far. It is quick and very cheap, but can be difficult to master, although in my experience the majority of doctors are able to handle it satisfactorily.

Electrical testing for food and chemical sensitivity

This method is based on the observation, repeatedly made when using intradermal injection techniques with dilutions of allergen concentrates, that when the so-called switch-off dilution is injected or placed sublingually, the patient's symptoms often disappear within seconds (hence the term 'switch-off'). This reaction is too quick for it to be mediated by a chemical mechanism and therefore an electrical change of an as yet ill-understood sort has been postulated. Electrical testing involves the use of this observation by applying a voltage to an acupuncture point (generally a terminal point is chosen on the fingers or toes) using a Wheatstone bridge circuit. The most commonly used technique uses the Vegatest device (Fig. 5.3). Either a food or chemical is placed in circuit, within a glass bottle. If the patient is sensitive to it, then the electrical reading over the acupuncture point changes. In skilled hands the success of this method is equal to that of all the other unconventional methods mentioned so far (i.e. 80%). It is cheap and quick and carries the added advantage of the placebo effect of a machine, which invariably maximises patient compliance, with an often rigorous dietary regime based upon the test results. The mechanism of action of this test is as yet unclear as it is not apparent as to why substances within a glass bottle should change impedance readings over acupuncture points, thus the observations noted are at variance with classical electromagnetic theory (Kenyon, in press).

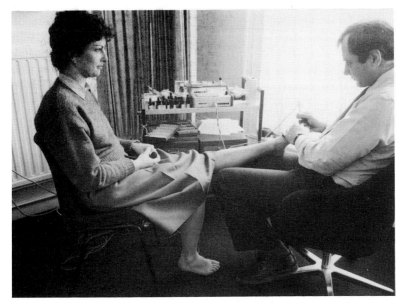

Fig. 5.3 The Vegatest method for detecting food and chemical sensitivities.

Applied kinesiology (muscle testing)

This method makes use of the observation that muscle power can be affected by placing a sensitive food or chemical either in the patient's hand or under the tongue as a sublingual drop. The mechanism of action is undoubtedly a change in the body field, much the same as in ACR and electrical testing. Its accuracy in skilled hands is again approximately 80%, but its disadvantage is that it is much more time consuming than either the ACR or electrical testing (Omura, 1979).

Conclusion

All the unconventional methods of testing are in-vivo techniques and are therefore much more applicable to the clinical situation. They are steadfastly resisted by conventional medicine as being unscientific, yet conventional techniques such as RAST have been shown to be ineffective clinically. The difference between conventional and unconventional testing methods in ecology goes to the core of the conceptual gap between conventional and alternative approaches to medicine. The alternative approach centres around the changes in biological energy and recording these in a whole-body sense, and by implication indicates that in-vitro tests of whatever sort are of limited relevance to the clinical situation which concerns the body as a whole, integrated and functioning unit. Any doctor wishing to practise ecology effectively would be well advised to learn and use a number of the alternative testing methods as these are the only approaches which will produce consistent and useful clinical results.

Ecological diagnosis enables the patient to follow a specific diet, and in clinical practice it is found that the diet is different in different patients for the same disease. This is of considerable importance as it means that it is impossible to devise a 'diet for arthritis' or a 'diet for colitis'. This therefore means that a testing method of some sort is essential. In many ways the advantages of an ecological approach are that the onus for the patient's illness lies very much with the patient rather than the doctor, and therefore the patient feels that he is doing something to help himself, and this often produces positive psychological changes in the patient's attitude to his problem. The ecological approach, however, does have dangers, the most common being that the patient is persuaded to follow a nutritionally inadequate diet for a long period of time which in the end results in a more chronically debilitated state than he was in before the diet was started. It is therefore very important to seek alternatives to the management of such patients and to look particularly for underlying causes for the multiple sensitivities.

Management of ecological illness

The simplest and most effective method of treatment is avoidance of the food and/or chemicals to which the patient has been found to be sensitive with whatever testing method has been used (*Food Intolerance and Food Aversion*, 1984, p. 36). With patients who are multiply food sensitive this can lead to nutritionally deficient diets which can become a serious problem in children. In these cases it is particularly important to look for underlying causes for their multiple sensitivities. A therapeutic approach based on the causal effects is more likely to prove effective in these patients. The services of a dietician with experience in ecology are invaluable in designing balanced diets for patients sensitive to commonly occurring foods such as milk, wheat or eggs, etc. The most important facts to know are the composition of commonly occurring composite foods (foods which contain a number of basic ingredients such as wheat and milk, etc.). Lists of commonly occurring foods are given in many ecology books (Rinkel *et al.*, 1951, Ch. 13), and are also in many books written for the lay public on diet and food-related illness.

Dangers of ecology diets

Severely restrictive ecological diets for patients, particularly children, have attracted much criticism because they are often nutritionally deficient. It is not uncommon to find a patient who has been eliminating milk and dairy products, wheat, corn and eggs, and has not received any proper dietary advice and, over a number of months, becomes nutritionally deficient and therefore less and less likely to respond to appropriate therapy, directed either at an underlying cause or at sorting the patient's diet out. This is a justified criticism of ecology and so emphasises the importance of having a balanced view when using an ecological approach. The technique most commonly used within ecology to get over this problem, that of sublingual desensitisation drops, also has its drawbacks. The main problems are that the patient tends to develop more and more sensitivities with the result that large numbers of 'switch-off' drops are accumulated. This, of itself, produces many psychological problems, with the patient often being frightened to eat, with again the result of a severely restricted and nutritionally inadequate diet. The practice of ecology which relies, to a major extent, on sublingual drop desensitisation restricts the use of ecology to the private sector, as these methods are very time consuming and enormously expensive, particularly as they rarely sort out any underlying problem which may be present

Rotation diets

Patients who have passed from the hyperacute sensitisation stage to the stage of latent sensitisation or tolerance can cope with the foods to which they are sensitive providing they are not included in the diet more than once in every 3 days. This therefore means that foods need to be eaten on a rotational basis (Rinkel *et al.*, 1951, Chs. 11 and 12). The periodicity of this rotation varies according to which authority is consulted, some recommending a 7-day rotation whereas others recommend a shorter cycle. In practice my experience has been that a 3-day rotation diet is adequate and practicable.

Desensitisation

This involves giving the patient sublingual drops of particular dilutions of the foods and/or chemicals to which they are sensitive (Miller, 1972). The specific dilutions necessary to switch reactions off are classically determined by the so-called Miller intradermal injection technique in which dilutions of the substances are injected intradermally (see page 201). Some practitioners follow this technique with unbounded enthusiasm, with the result that patients may receive as many as 50 'switch-off' drops to various foods and chemicals. In a proportion of patients this technique does work, but it has a number of serious drawbacks. The first and most troublesome is that sublingual drop desensitisation often leads to the development of new sensitivities to other foods and chemicals. The implication is that the patient's problem is due to an underlying cause which has not been identified, the food and chemical sensitivities being an effect of that cause. Therefore in many ways this technique is not ideal, but in some cases provides a convenient method for allowing the patient to eat out, or go away on holiday, or be able to live a normal sort of life. Its main disadvantages are that finding the 'end-points' (the so-called switch-off dilutions) using the classical method is, as has already been mentioned, time consuming and consequently expensive. From a psychological point of view it is often detrimental to the patient as it leads him to excessive and in many cases harmful introspection. The ACR and electrical testing methods offer two much quicker ways of finding the end-points. In my view the use of sublingual dilutions for the 'switch-offs' has a limited application only in food and chemical sensitivity.

Underlying causes of multiple food and chemical sensitivity

Most cases who are severely multiply sensitive to foods and/or chemicals are so because of an underlying problem. The key to treating these patients is recognising this problem and coping with it satisfactorily. The most common underlying problems are as follows (in order of frequency of occurrence).

1. *Dysbiosis.* Dysbiosis means colonic dysfunction, most commonly due to abnormal colonic flora. The integrity of the gastrointestinal mucous membrane has been shown to be central to the normal tolerance of foods. If this is significantly disturbed, then the patient's gastrointestinal mucosa behaves like a sieve in which the holes are too big. As a consequence, peptides instead of amino acids are absorbed. These peptides are often highly active in the body and produce a wide range of symptoms seen in ecological illness. It is of some interest to note that the vast majority of patients with ecological illness have symptoms connected with the gastrointestinal tract. Treatment of the dysbiosis is therefore central to enabling the patient to recover normal tolerance of foods. This has been outlined in detail elsewhere (Kenyon, in press) and centres around the use of a combination of naturopathic dietary approaches (in simple terms this involves a low-fat, low-carbohydrate, non-processed food diet) and complex homoeopathy.

2. *Post-viral states.* Severe viral illnesses, particularly influenza and glandular fever, seem to upset the body's immune defences and as a result many patients become multiply sensitive. The key to treatment is recognising the underlying cause of post-viral debility and treating this. In my experience the most successful approach has been found to be complex homoeopathy (Kenyon, in press).

3. *Toxicity.* Poisoning of any sort, whether acute or, more commonly, chronic insidious poisoning, can be the cause of multiple sensitivity (Kenyon, in press). Diagnosing this problem can be exceptionally difficult, and to date electrical techniques as used in complex homoeopathy (Kenyon, in press) constitute the only practicable approaches. The treatment involves avoiding continued exposure, and removal of the toxin from the patient's tissues. The only successful method of achieving this, in my experience to date, has been using an appropriate homoeopathic nosode (a homoeopathic dilution of a substance which in its concentrated form is pathogenic, in this case a toxin) together with appropriate homoeopathic accompanying remedies.

4. *Psychological causes.* A number of multiply food- and chemical-sensitive patients have an underlying psychological

cause to their problem which can be difficult to recognise and may be missed by the enthusiastic ecologist who sees himself as being a haven from the psychiatrist. Patients with psychological problems are all too ready to take up the ecologist's offer of help as it avoids them having to sort out their underlying problems. A sensible and carefully judged approach is therefore essential on the part of every practitioner to be able to recognise these cases.

Conclusion

Ecology has tended to develop into a specialty of its own, particularly in America, with the consequence that ecological illness is looked at in a narrow sense. The result is that underlying causes are rarely recognised and that many multiply sensitive patients are being managed with narrow and highly inappropriate regimes. This is a prime example of the dangers of specialisation seen most glaringly within conventional medicine but here alas occurring also within alternative medicine. It is to be hoped that the lesson provided by ecology will be well learnt by those practitioners who read this book.

Chemical sensitivity

Chemical sensitivity has until recently been the Cinderella of ecology. In clinical terms chemical sensitivity is at least as important, if not more important, in many patients with food sensitivity. Clinical evidence from everyday practice indicates that many patients are sensitive to commercially produced wheat but are able to eat organically produced wheat, implying that the chemical adulteration of commercially grown crops with insecticides, pesticides and fertilizers, etc. is a possible cause of the commonly occurring sensitivities to these foods.

Chemical sensitivity has been the subject of a number of lay books which variously predict Armageddon within the foreseeable future (Mackarness, 1980). In practice all that is required is the creation of a safe haven for the patient to live in, free of the worst pollutants, and a balanced view of the dangers of chemical sensitivity. Some ecology books provide such a balanced view (Lewith and Kenyon, in press). The most important sources of chemical sensitivity are as follows.

1. Hydrocarbons (petrol, diesel, gas, fuel oil, etc.).
2. Formaldehyde.
3. Phenol.

Many other chemical sensitivities do occur but are not as common as the above. The incidence of sensitivity to food additives is not as high as popularly thought (*Food Intolerance and Food Aversion*, 1984, pp. 30-32), but the general recommendation that the patient sticks to a diet as free as possible from processed foods remains wise.

Hydrocarbon sensitivity

Patients with hydrocarbon sensitivity often complain of what the Americans call 'brain fag'. This describes an intermittent state of varying severity (depending on the degree of sensitivity and the level of exposure) of mental confusion, poor memory, slurring of speech and a general dulling of all the senses. The clue as to the cause of these problems comes from the history. For example, the patient who goes to sleep sitting in front of the gas fire or near to a mobile calor gas heater, but does not become so affected when sitting in front of an electric fire; or the patient who suffers from car sickness; the motorist who constantly has to fight extreme fatigue when motorway driving: all these suggest hydrocarbon sensitivity.

It should be remembered that we are surrounded by a vast number of hydrocarbon derivatives, particularly plastics. Patients must be screened for hydrocarbon sensitivity and, if sensitive, must have them removed in so far as it is possible from their immediate environment.

Formaldehyde sensitivity

Formalin is similar to hydrocarbons in that its use is widespread and people are very often sensitive to it. It is contained in many different products, often in unexpected places. For example, it is a degradation product of foam backing from cheap carpets (Tucker, 1984). It is also released from urea formaldehyde foam cavity wall insulation (this form of home insulation has now been banned in Canada due to resultant health problems). Diagnosis of formaldehyde sensitivity is often extremely difficult and can rarely be made on clinical grounds alone. A testing technique is essential in order to identify this problem.

Phenol sensitivity

Phenol, like formaldehyde and hydrocarbons, is a ubiquitous substance. It is a commonly used preservative in medications and is found in nylon and polyurethane. Many household cleaning materials contain phenol. The same comments apply as to formaldehyde.

The diagnosis of multiple chemical sensitivity is difficult for the beginner in ecology to make. Testing for the most commonly occurring hydrocarbons (petrol, diesel and gas) as well as phenol and formaldehyde should be a mandatory part of any ecological screen. Management is best carried out by avoiding the offending chemicals. In many cases this is impossible to achieve totally and can only be managed partially, and then the use of the sublingual drop desensitisation method using the Miller technique (Miller, 1972) comes into its own. In multiply chemically sensitive patients the identification of an underlying cause and its successful treatment become of major importance.

The observant doctor will undoubtedly recognise the most obvious form of chemical sensitivity in many of his patients, that of drug reaction. It is hoped that such reactions will have been sufficiently obvious to have been eliminated as a cause of the presenting symptoms. This often gives a clue as to the underlying ecological problem in a patient who shows multiple drug reactions.

Conclusion

Clinical ecology is a useful discipline for managing a wide range of clinical problems. It is of considerable importance that it is not followed in a narrow fashion but in a critical and open-minded way. With this approach, severely sensitive patients will not have to commit themselves to the 'ecology merry-go-round', but rather will have their problems dealt with in a sensible and appropriate manner. The mechanisms underlying multiple food and chemical sensitivity still elude us but are likely to be due to energetic changes in the body produced by offending foods and/or chemicals. It is highly likely that cell-mediated immunity has a major part to play in the mediation of these reactions. A more broad-minded approach to research is therefore necessary if we are to learn anything more clinically useful about this interesting approach to disease.

Where do interested practitioners go from here?

This chapter should be regarded as an introduction to ecology.

Due to reasons of space, many aspects of ecology, particularly chemical sensitivity, have not been dealt with in depth. Topics related to ecology, such as Candida sensitivity and hair analysis for vitamin and mineral balance and heavy metal poisoning, have not been mentioned at all. Any therapist interested in learning how to use ecology would be well advised to attend a training course on the subject. To date, very few have been available in the United Kingdom but many have been taking place in the United States for some years. Typically, the American courses tend to be orientated towards a particular approach to ecology, such as ecological desensitisation using dilutions. In the United Kingdom a group of doctors interested in ecology has recently formed the Clinical Ecology Society, which regards it as one of its functions to teach ecology to interested doctors. This society runs one course a year and two scientific meetings; generally these are held in London.

A wider ranging course open to doctors and paramedical professions is run by the Centre for the Study of Alternative Therapies, Southampton. This course attempts to teach all of the useful approaches to ecology, both from a conventional and from an unconventional standpoint. The aim is to turn out a practitioner who can confidently handle an ecological approach to common clinical problems.

References

Abboton D. J. (1982). Atopic eczema. *Clinics in Immunology and Allergy*; 2:77–100.

Anderson G. M. (1981). Diet, neurotransmitters and brain function. *British Medical Bulletin*; 37:95–100.

Barnetson R. St. C., Lessof M. H. (1983). Challenges to medical orthodoxy. In *Clinical Reactions to Food* (Lessof M. H., ed.) pp. 15–34. Chichester: J. Wiley.

Black A. P. (1956). A new diagnostic method in allergic disease. *Paediatrics*; 17:716–24.

Breneman J. C., Hurst A., Heiner D., Leney F. L., Morris D., Josephson B. M. (1974). Final report of the Food Allergy Committee of the American College of Allergists on the clinical evaluation of sublingual provocative testing method for diagnosis of food allergy. *Annals of Allergy*; 33:164–6.

Committee on Provocative Food Testing (1973). *Annals of Allergy*; 31: 375–81.

Cooke W. T., Holmes G. K. T. (1983). Coeliac disease, inflammatory bowel disease and food intolerance. In *Clinical Reactions to Food* (Lessof M. H., ed.) p. 187. Chichester: J. Wiley.

Denman A. M. (1983). Food allergy. Leading article. *British Medical Journal*; 286: 1164–6.

Dohan F. C. (1966). Cereals and schizophrenia: data and hypothesis. *Acta Psychiatrica Scandinavica*; 42:125–52.

Dong C. H., Banks J. (1976). *New Hope for the Arthritic*. London: Hart-Davis, MacGibbon.

Egger J., Carter C. M., Wilson J., Turner M. W., Soothill J. F. (1983). Is migraine food allergy? A double-blind controlled trial of oligoantigenic diet treatment. *Lancet*; 2:865–9.

Ferguson A., Strobel S. (1983). Immunology and physiology of digestion. In *Clinical Reactions to Food* (Lessof M. H., ed.) pp. 59–86. Chichester: J. Wiley.

Ferguson A., Strobel S., Hanson D. G., Pickering M. G. (1983). Regulation of immune responses to a fed protein antigen. In *The Second Fisons Food Allergy Workshop*, pp. 1–4. Oxford: Medicine Publishing Foundation.

Ferriman A. (1983). Clinic fails its own allergy test. *Observer*; 3rd April.

Freed D. L. J. (1983). Antibodies in migraine. In *The Second Fisons Food Allergy Workshop*, pp. 135–6. Oxford: Medicine Publishing Foundation.

Food Intolerance and Food Aversion. (1984). Joint Report of the Royal College of Physicians and the British Nutrition Foundation. Reprinted from the *Journal of the Royal College of Physicians*; 18 (2).

Grant G., More L. J., McKenzie N. H., Steward J. C., Pusztai A. (1983). A survey of the nutritional and haemagglutination properties of legume seeds generally available in the UK. *British Journal of Nutrition*; 50:207–14.

Hanington E. (1983). Migraine. In *Clinical Reactions to Food* (Lessof M. H., ed.) pp. 155–80. Chichester: J. Wiley.

Haverberg L., Kwon T. H., Scrimshaw N. S. (1980). Comparative tolerance of adolescents of differing ethnic backgrounds to lactose-containing and lactose-free dairy drinks. Initial experience with a double blind procedure. *American Journal of Clinical Nutrition*; 33:17–21.

Hunter J. O., Alun-Jones V., Freeman A. J., Shorthouse N., Workman E., McLaughlan P. (1983). Food intolerance in gastrointestinal disorders. In *The Second Fisons Food Allergy Workshop*, pp. 69–72. Oxford: Medicine Publishing Foundation.

Jackson D., Phillips A.D., Haidas A., Walker-Smith J. A. (1983). Morphological studies of the small intestine in children with food intolerance and related problems. In *The Second Fisons Food Allergy Workshop*, pp. 10–17. Oxford: Medicine Publishing Foundation.

Jakobsson I., Lindberg T. (1978). Cow's milk as a cause of infantile colic in breast fed infants. *Lancet*; 2:437–9.

Juhlin L. (1981). Recurrent urticaria: clinical investigation of 330 patients. *British Journal of Dermatology*; 104:369–81.

Keneny D. M., Parkes P., Lessof M. H. (1983). Setting up RAST to measure IgE antibodies to foods. In *The Second Fisons Food Allergy Workshop*, pp. 45–7. Oxford: Medicine Publishing Foundation.

Kenyon J. N. (1983). *Modern Techniques of Acupuncture*, Vol. II. Wellingborough: Thorsons.

Kenyon J. N. (in press). *Modern Techniques of Acupuncture*, Vol. III. Wellingborough: Thorsons.

Leading article (1979). Feingold's regimen for hyperkinesis. *Lancet*; 2:617–18.

Lessof M. H. (1983). Reactions to food in adults. In *Clinical Reactions to Food* (Lessof M. H., ed.) pp. 103–33. Chichester: J. Wiley.

Lewith G. T., Kenyon J. N. (in press). *Clinical Ecology*. Wellingborough: Thorsons.

Mackarness R. (1961). *Eat Fat and Grow Slim*. London: Fontana.

Mackarness R. (1976). *Not all in the Mind*. London: Pan.

Mackarness R. (1980). *Chemical Victims*. London: Pan.

Miller J. B. (1972). *Food Allergy*. Springfield, Illinois: Charles C Thomas.

Mitchell E. B., Crow J., Chapman M. D., Jouhal S. S., Pope F. M., Platts-Mills T. A. E. (1982). Basophils in allergen-induced patch test sites in atopic dermatitis. *Lancet*; 1:127–30.

Moneret-Vautrin D. A. (1983). False food allergies. Non-specific reactions to food stuffs. In *Clinical Reactions to Food* (Lessof M. H., ed.) pp. 148–9. Chichester: J. Wiley.

Ogle K. A., Bullock J. D. (1977). Children with allergic rhinitis and/or bronchial asthma treated with elimination diet. *Annals of Allergy*; 39:8–11.

Omura Y. (1979). Applied kinesiology using the acupuncture meridian concept: critical evaluation of its potential as the simplest non-invasive means of diagnosis, and compatibility test of food and drugs. Part I. *Acupuncture and Electro-Therapeutics Reasearch, the International Journal*; 4 (3):165–84.

Rinkel H. J., Randolph T. G., Zeller N. (1951). *Food Allergy*. Springfield, Illinois: Charles C Thomas.

Rosen S. N., Bennett M. K., Faux J., Jewell D. P. (1983). Chronic gastritis—an allergic disorder? In *The Second Fisons Food Allergy Workshop*, pp. 73–6. Oxford: Medicine Publishing Foundation.

Skoldstam L., Larsson L., Lindstrom F. D. (1979). Effects of fasting and lacto-vegetarian diet on rheumatoid arthritis. *Scandinavian Journal of Rheumatology*; 8:249–55.

Soothill J. F., Harries J. T., Jenkins H. R., Millar P. J., Pincott J. R. (1983). Food allergy in infantile colitis. In *The Second Fisons Food Allergy Workshop*, pp. 77–8. Oxford: Medicine Publishing Foundation.

Stenius B. S. M., Lemola M. (1976). Hypersensitivity to acetylsalicylic acid (ASA) and tartrazine in patients with asthma. *Clinical Allergy*; 6:119–29.

Tucker A. (1984). The built-in dangers. *Guardian*, p. 13, 3rd May.

Vedanthan T. K., Menon M. M., Bell T. D., Bergin D. J. (1977). Aspirin and tartrazine oral challenge: incidence of adverse response in chronic childhood asthma. *Journal of Allergy and Clinical Immunology*; 60: 8–13.

Walport M. H., Parke A. L., Hughes G. V. (1983). Food and the connective tissue diseases. In *Food Allergy* (Prostoff J., Challacomb S. J., eds.) pp. 113–20. London: Saunders.

For those practitioners wishing to read further on the subject of ecology, many books are available. Most are American and suffer from a common drawback of many American textbooks in that they could all be condensed to a quarter of the space and not lose anything in factual content. An excellent booklist is available from Action Against Allergy, 43 The Downs, London SW20. The best books are as follows.

For the lay reader

Lewith G. T., Kenyon J. N. (in press). *Clinical Ecology*. Wellingborough: Thorsons.

For the professional reader

Dickey L. (ed.) (1976). *Clinical Ecology*. Springfield, Illinois: Charles C Thomas.

Lessof M. H. (ed.) (1983). *Clinical Reactions to Food*. Chichester: J. Wiley.

Miller J. B. (1972). *Food Allergy, Provocative Testing and Injection Therapy*. Springfield, Illinois: Charles C Thomas.

Rinkel H. J., Randolph T. G., Zeller N. (1951). *Food Allergy*. Springfield, Illinois: Charles C Thomas.

Rowe A. H. (1972). *Food Allergy, Its Manifestations and Control and the Elimination Diets, a Compendium.* Springfield, Illinois: Charles C Thomas.

Useful addresses

Secretary of the Clinical Ecology Society
Dr J. Mansfield
Burghwood Clinic
34 Brighton Road
Banstead
Surrey SM7 3HH.

The Centre for the Study of Alternative Therapies
51 Bedford Place
Southampton SO1 2DG.

Action Against Allergy
Head Office
43 The Downs
London SW20 8HG.
(This is an informal society whose members suffer from food and chemical sensitivity.)

British Society for Nutritional Medicine
c/o Dr S. Davies (Chairman)
9 Portland Road
East Grimstead
West Sussex RH19 4EB.

Index